I have known Matt for almost ten years now and [illegible] ard him as a compliant patient with the drive to make a [illegible] g others with lymphoedema.

Now, he is making new ground [illegible] has ever been done in this way before, as [illegible] again, I think provides a unique service to peop[illegible] am very pleased to have been Matt's sounding board, a[illegible] e him with support and encouragement along the way.

—Prof. Peter Mortimer MD, FRCP
Professor of Dermatological Medicine

I have supported Matt on his journey to secure a diagnosis and long-term management plan for his lymphoedema. I suspect Matt will agree that it has been a journey filled with highs and occasional lows. I believe we have learnt a great deal from each other, both about an individual's response to lymphoedema treatment and the psychological impact this disease can inflict.

I look forward to continuing to support Matt with managing his lymphoedema for many more years and am optimistic that the future of lymphoedema care will continue to develop and improve.

—Dr Kristiana Gordon MBBS, CLT, MD(Res), FRCP
Consultant in Dermatology and Lymphovascular Medicine

I am very honoured to be invited to be part of your project and delighted to be able to accept.

—Prof. Vaughan Keeley PhD, FRCP
Consultant in Lymphoedema

I was delighted when Matt asked me to contribute to this book, and his forthcoming website. I truly believe that only by informing the patient of all options available to them can they make a fully informed decision about their care. Too often, patients have come to me asking why their doctor or practitioner didn't inform them of our surgical service years ago, leaving them to suffer in isolation. It is only through initiatives like this that patients can be empowered.

—Prof. Dominic Furniss DM MA MBBCh FRCS(Plast)
Professor of Plastic and Reconstructive Surgery

Matt and I have been involved in a torrent of emails fuelled by his determination to be a game-changer in this quickly evolving field of lymphatic disease (LD). The fact that Matt lives with lymphedema (LE) was of particular interest to me. I am always looking for the leaders who will forge the changes needed before LDs and LE become global priorities.

The bond that ensued from our likeminded curiosity and determination led to Matt asking me to write a chapter for this book. I do so with pleasure and as prologue to what I envision as Matt's future impact on this field.

—William Repicci
President & CEO, Lymphatic Education & Research Network (LE&RN)

Matt was very keen from the outset to see how he could help the LSN. Matt had a particular interest in raising awareness of lymphoedema, particularly among men who live with primary forms of the condition, he was ultimately invited to join the LSN Trustee Board, focussing on our corporate relationships and fundraising.

We know that raising awareness among men remains Matt's passion and we wish him every success in his new ventures.

—Chair, Lymphoedema Support Network (LSN)

I had the opportunity to engage Matt as a consultant when Haddenham Healthcare were looking to build a patient focused retail platform for lymphoedema patients. Matt's diligent work ethic, business knowledge and passion for empowering lymphoedema patients was invaluable in helping to deliver a successful project.

—Tom Wright
Director, Haddenham Healthcare Ltd

There are many gaps in provision of care, support and knowledge in relation to lymphoedema and Matt had certainly identified with some of these through his own harrowing experiences. Filling these gaps needs a multidimensional approach and for all of us who are passionate about doing so to collaborate. I am delighted that Matt and the BLS are continuing discussions about how we can work together effectively and am honoured to be invited to contribute to this book.

—Margaret Sneddon
Chair, British Lymphology Society

I have known of Matt's work within the lymphoedema community for a number of years. His willingness to share the story of his own lymphoedema, including his experiences with lymph node transfer and liposuction surgery, with others is admirable and I immediately loved his idea to write this book, particularly because it is written specifically for the patient, for the individual living with, and so often struggling with, the condition that is lymphoedema, on a day-to-day basis. I am confident that this book will give you an introduction to the many treatments and protocols that you may have heard mentioned, but not known where to access more facts, data and statistics.

—Naomi Northen-Ellis
Director, Compression Therapy UK Ltd

Matt was desperately trying to find solutions and asked many questions that I couldn't answer, including surgical options. I did some bandaging (MLLB) but I knew he needed long-term care.

—Mark Pearson
MLD Therapist & Paediatric and Primary Lymphoedema Clinic Coordinator

In the time I have been running L-W-O Community I have met many amazing people all of whom are passionate about the lymphoedema community. I was introduced to Matt Hazledine at the LSN Conference at Edgbaston in 2018 and have since spoken on the phone and exchanged several emails. I am delighted to contribute to his book and support the work he does to inform and educate those of us who live with lymphoedema.

—Gaynor Leech
Founder, Lymph-What-Oedema Community

I am delighted and feel very honoured to be involved with your book Matt, which I know is going to be a great success.

—Rebecca Elwell Msc Lymphoedema
Macmillan Lymphoedema ANP and Team Leader & BLS Trustee

I will never forget seeing Matt walk into Levi's in his Lot 1's. Every inch of him stood tall and proud, and he certainly had a swagger. It's not often with tailoring that one can feel they really made a difference, but I know that these jeans have for Matt and I am immensely proud that with this service we can problem solve whilst creating beautiful jeans too!

—Elizabeth Radcliffe
Master Tailor, Levi's Lot 1

How to LIVE BETTER with LYMPHOEDEMA

Meet the Experts

Personal experiences and tips from someone living with lymphoedema, combined with trusted information and helpful guidance from medical professionals in the lymphoedema sector

"I wish I'd had this book 10 years ago, when I was diagnosed with lymphoedema"

Matt Hazledine & Guests

First published 2021 by Wordzworth Publishing

ISBN: 978-1-78324-220-7 (paperback)
ISBN: 978-1-78324-221-4 (ebook)

Book design and typesetting by *www.wordzworth.com*

Dedicated to my fantastic wife and best friend, Vicki; my beautiful daughters, Amber and Jasmine; my wonderful, selfless parents, Annie & Roy; my supportive sister, Sam; and all my close friends. I am truly blessed to have you all in my life and sincerely appreciate your continued love and support.

Thank you to Professor Peter Mortimer for the generosity of his time, support and encouragement with my lymphoedema projects, in addition to his expert care and advice over the years.

Thank you to all of the amazingly talented experts for their informative and beneficial contributions in this book, and for their unconditional care during my journey with lymphoedema so far.

CONTENTS

FOREWORD

Lymphoedema is a debilitating disease that can have a detrimental effect on both the physical and mental wellbeing of the sufferer. Living with this lifelong condition can be incredibly challenging and often lonely. It is a daunting task trying to find expert help and information.

This book has been devised and edited by Matt Hazledine, a sufferer of lymphoedema, who has had a very difficult time, not of his making, in overcoming this disease. The book provides a comprehensive and especially helpful one-stop-shop approach to the key elements of living with lymphoedema presented in a novel, practical format. Covering over 30 subjects, the chapters are perfectly balanced as Matt articulately shares his personal experiences of living with lymphoedema since 2011 as well as providing many useful tips throughout the book. This is combined with comprehensive information and authoritative advice from over 20 medical professionals and lymphoedema experts, many of whom are recognised globally for their knowledge and expertise.

Thanks to increased awareness, more people are being correctly diagnosed with lymphoedema, although there is still a long way to go before lymphoedema and other lymphatic diseases become well recognised by most doctors. The decline in the number of specialist lymphoedema therapists has made it even more important for patients with lymphoedema to be informed and knowledgeable about their condition. It is vital that patients learn from the professionals' self-management recommendations to control their swelling and better manage their health.

I have known Matt since 2012 and can honestly say, I regard him as a model patient with the drive to make a positive contribution by helping others with lymphoedema. He is breaking new ground in creating this book and producing a new website, which I think provides a unique service to people living with lymphoedema.

Matt is very passionate about making a positive difference and helping others with the condition, to live better with lymphoedema and I am very pleased to provide him with my support and encouragement along the way.

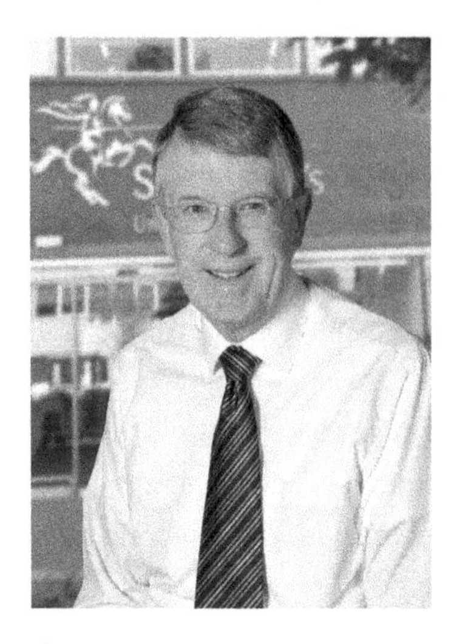

Professor Peter Mortimer MD, FRCP

PREFACE
WHY HAVE I WRITTEN THIS BOOK NOW?

This is an easy one. If, by reading this book, you discover just one piece of information, or a useful tip that improves your quality of life and wellbeing, then I have achieved my objective which is to help you to live better with lymphoedema.

At the point of writing, I approach the 10-year anniversary of being diagnosed with this chronic condition (disease) back in June 2011. Since then, it is fair to say that I have experienced practically all compression aids, treatments, therapies and surgeries available to man, all of which have assisted *me* in *my* journey to live better with lymphoedema. Although, I can only speak about my personal experiences, the content in this book is relevant to anyone who suffers from lymphoedema and those supporting a loved one with the condition.

So, what better way to mark the anniversary than to write a book, share my story and provide some 40 useful tips along the way. I am honoured to feature trusted information and helpful guidance from 23 guests, including specialist healthcare professionals and industry experts, for whom I have tremendous respect. These wonderful human beings have been, and in many cases will continue to be, instrumental in making my lifelong journey with lymphoedema as comfortable as possible, whilst having a positive impact on my wellbeing. I am very grateful for their ongoing care and support.

I share my story with you to provide positivity and hope. This is not my platform to moan about how unfair life is and 'why me?,' which to be fair, I no doubt did in the first year or so of having lymphoedema. During the first few months following my diagnosis, I felt lost and abandoned by the healthcare system. This affected me physically and mentally, until, thanks to my fabulous wife Vicki, we found the help I so desperately needed, guiding me to a much better place all round.

I hope my story will resonate with you in some way and demonstrate to you that I have walked the walk and therefore am qualified, if only as a patient, to talk the talk.

Before we begin, I would like to state that I am not a medical expert in any way, shape or form and I am not qualified to provide you with medical advice or guidance. The content written by all the guest medical professionals and experts has not been edited in any way.

If you have any medical related questions about your oedema, please contact your GP or a qualified lymphoedema therapist.

What I can do, is talk confidently and with comprehensive experience of being a person who lives with this lifelong condition called lymphoedema (or lymphedema if you are American).

My book coincides with the launch of *www.lymphoedemaunited.com* a free membership website that connects people living with lymphoedema with a panel of medical experts, organisations, charities and a virtual shopping centre with specialist product suppliers. Please sign up as a free member to receive regular newsletters and unique member's benefits. You can also follow us at @LymphUnited, which is available on most popular social media platforms. In addition, we will launch the new 'Lymphoedema United Support Group' also under the name of LymphUnited on Facebook. Check our website and social media for details.

I am committed to donate **25%** of pre-tax profits raised from the sales of this book to the Lymphoedema Research Fund, managed by St George's Hospital Charity. Thank you for buying this book and making a positive contribution to medical research with the aim of finding a cure for lymphoedema.

"I wish I'd had this book 10 years ago, when I was diagnosed with lymphoedema."

MEDICAL ADVICE DISCLAIMER

This Book Does Not Provide Medical Advice

All material in this book is for informational purposes only and is not a substitute for professional medical advice, diagnosis or treatment.

Always seek the advice of your physician or other qualified healthcare provider with any questions you may have regarding a medical condition or treatment and before undertaking a new health care regime. Never disregard professional medical advice or delay in seeking it because of something you have read in this book.

Reliance on any information provided in this book by the author and others featured in the book is solely at your own risk.

Any information and guidance written in this book by any medical expert, organisation or guest has not been edited in any way by the author. Content written by the author, is done so in the context of providing insights as a person living with lymphoedema since 2011 and should not be considered as medical advice in any capacity.

For the avoidance of any doubt, Matt Hazledine has lymphoedema and is not a medical professional.

Authenticity of Content

It is important to note that any content written by my guests has not been changed or edited in any way and therefore, I do not take any responsibility for the accuracy of the information provided.

To ensure that the book is authentic and honest, I can assure you that all content written by me, has not been edited by an expert ghost writer or a publisher. It is from my heart, frank in places, but always with the intention of helping others who live with lymphoedema.

All prices quoted in the book are in GBP and correct at the time of going to print.

Matt Hazledine

1

INTRODUCTION

If you have lymphoedema or know someone who does, this book will provide invaluable information from the experts and useful tips to help you better manage the condition, improving your quality of life and mental wellbeing.

When I was diagnosed with lymphoedema, some of the biggest problems for me were where to go for expert care, support, information and advice. This book contains everything and everyone I wish I knew from the point of diagnosis, rather than being left to my own devices.

I share 10 years of personal experiences, solutions to problems, provide 40 tips, cover over 30 relevant topics and introduce you to over 20 experts all in one book, which I hope you find helpful and informative. We cover the four cornerstones of treatment: Compression, Skin Care, Healthy Lifestyle & Movement and Lymphatic Drainage, in addition to tackling the effect lymphoedema can have on mental health and wellbeing. You can read it from front to back and/or refer to specific chapters as they become relevant to your personal circumstances.

I can honestly say that by applying the expert advice provided to me over the years, I am back to the confident, healthy, outgoing person I was before lymphoedema. As you will read, it has been a very bumpy and winding road with numerous highs and lows. I am confident that you will benefit from this book now and in the future, and that the information provided will help you to control the lymphoedema, rather than letting the lymphoedema control you.

This book *will* help *you* to live better with lymphoedema *and* raise money for the Lymphoedema Research Fund to help find a cure.

The Day My Life Changed, Forever

Saturday 18th June 2011, the day before Father's Day. My wife and two-year-old daughter were excited to take me to the American Golf shop for me to choose a new putter, as my Father's Day gift. I had received the current putter as a present for my 16th birthday, so at the age of 40 it was probably time to get a new one, hopefully one that worked better and holed more putts! On leaving the shop with my new golf club in hand we drove the thirty-minute journey home. En route, we stopped off at the local supermarket to pick up a nice dinner, (rather than a horrible one) before settling in for the afternoon playing games and watching a film.

Whilst waiting in the car with my daughter, I suddenly felt unwell, which came quite literally from nowhere. I was freezing cold and shivering, a bit like proper old fashioned flu symptoms. On arriving home, I couldn't even help to unload the shopping as I had to try and warm up under my duvet. Within 20 minutes, I was lying curled up convulsing, unusually cold, with sweats. It was pretty scary, especially as it had come totally out of the blue. I had a hot bath, but that had no effect on how cold I was feeling. It transpired that I had a temperature of over 40°C. Apparently, by now I was a bit delirious and my now, very concerned wife Vicki, decided to take me to A&E, leaving our daughter with a friend.

The next memory I have is curling up in a side room of the A&E Department of Maidstone Hospital, my body shaking and feeling oblivious to anything around me. As a fit and healthy 40-year-old, just under 6'4", this hit me like a ton of bricks and so quickly too. I was moved to a side room and given morphine to help with the pain and it wasn't long before I was being admitted to a ward and put under observation. The initial diagnosis was an infection and I was prescribed intravenous antibiotics. However, it was many hours before I received the antibiotics because the staff were rushed off their feet.

I soon became aware of a small red rash on my left shin, about the size of a 5p piece. It was hot and itchy and became very painful as it spread incredibly rapidly, covering my complete lower leg before moving to my thigh, literally within a few hours of being admitted. I had never seen anything like it before and never experienced such excruciating pain. When standing to visit the bathroom, the pain was so intense that I had to use a walking frame and take pigeon steps. It felt as though acid was being poured down my leg, a pain I will never forget to this day and I do have a high pain threshold.

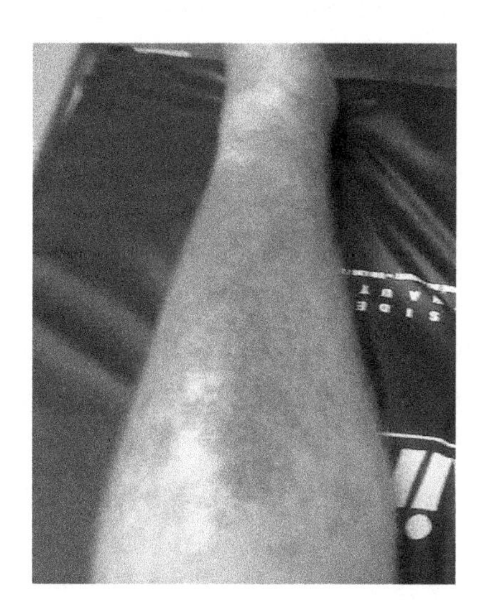

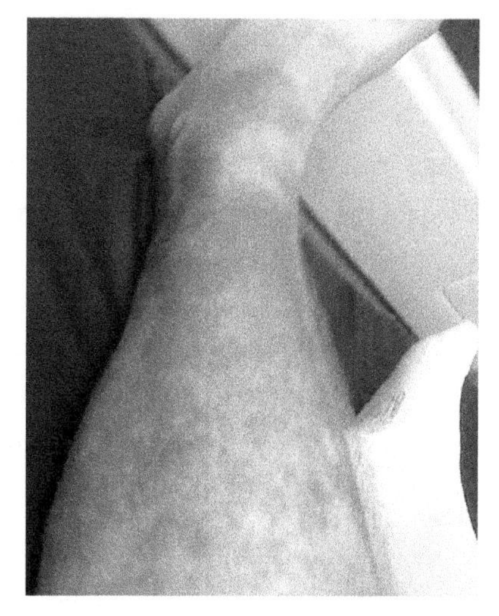

Cellulitis in Matt's left leg - June 2011

Two days later, I was waiting for the blood culture test results to come back when a doctor came to see me. She asked if I'd yet had an X-ray, which I hadn't and I asked why I needed one. My wife was with me at the time when the doctor said they needed to rule out necrotising fasciitis. On asking what that was, Vicki responded with, 'isn't that flesh-eating disease?' which it is. I probed further as to what that would mean and was told that if I have it, I may require amputation. At that point in time, the world stood still. All I could think about were the challenges of living as an amputee. I had a wife, two young daughters and a new business venture that was only launched six months previously. This came as a terrifying shock. After being rushed down for an X-ray, the next two hours waiting for the results seemed like an eternity, with millions of 'What if' thoughts running through my head. Thankfully, the X-ray results were negative and this frightening condition was ruled out, much to our immense relief.

Later that day, the blood cultures showed that there were Staphylococcus and Streptococcus bacteria present, and I was then diagnosed with an infection called cellulitis. It appeared that the bacteria may have entered via an open blister on my little toe, caused by wearing brand new golf shoes.

Now that the infection had been correctly identified, I was immediately put on a cocktail of intravenous and oral antibiotics, with a side order of painkillers including the odd hit of Oramorph when the pain was at its height. Despite the doctor confirming that the combination of antibiotics was equivalent to 'bleach', it took five days for my temperature to come down.

I spent 13 nights and 14 long days in hospital, cared for by some wonderful nurses. During my second week, my leg started to swell, quite noticeably, from foot to thigh, which raised much concern. None of the medical staff seemed to know why or what it was. Later that week I was visited by a Consultant Vascular Surgeon, who told me, very bluntly, that I now had a lifelong disease called lymphoedema. I was told to see the Supplies Team for a stocking before being discharged. And that was that. The total extent of the explanation that I received. I was grateful that Vicki was there to hear it too. A stocking? What is this disease? What is the treatment? How long would my leg be swollen for? Where do I go for help? I received nothing, nada, nichts, rien, absolutely nowt!

I received two off the shelf circular knit stockings from the Supplies Team and when asking if I could get more, the reply was a huge sigh, followed by 'you'll have to ask your GP.' That was the magnitude of the aftercare at that early stage of diagnosis. I left hospital on day 14 about to face the unknown.

I want to make it clear that, from arrival in A&E, to the day I was discharged, I could not fault the care and compassion that I had received during my stay. It ended with appreciative hugs with a few of the outstanding nurses with whom I had bonded. It was only from discharge and the very awkward conversation with the Supplies Team, that I remember feeling abandoned. This sounds very dramatic now but please bear in mind that this was in 2011 and aftercare for cellulitis/lymphoedema patients has hopefully improved significantly since then.

Lymphoedema is a disease that is with me for life. The first few months after diagnosis (OK who am I kidding - the first year) were an incredibly difficult time for me and my family, and in fact probably my biggest low point ever. However, I can look back now and draw on my experiences to help others living with lymphoedema, by sharing useful tips and introducing them to the experts.

I am extremely grateful to have been treated by some of the most accredited medical professionals in this field over the years, all with the NHS, and I am honoured that many of them have contributed to my book. I am also very thankful to those people who have been involved in any way along my winding road. Lymphoedema-Land really feels like an inclusive and supportive community and I am blessed to have made so many friendships in the medical sector and beyond.

During the chapters ahead, I continue to share my experiences pertinent to the subject in question, whilst introducing many medical professionals who impart their knowledge and guidance. In addition, they respond to questions that every person with lymphoedema wants to know the answers to.

You may have noticed that I have already referred to lymphoedema as both a condition and as a disease. Such is the strength of opinion on how to classify lymphoedema, I have dedicated a sub-chapter to this very subject 'Condition or Disease?.'

I hope you gain some benefit from this book. There is much, much more to cover and I was thinking of naming some of the chapters: 'Help! I need somebody,' 'Blue Jeans,' 'A cut above the rest' and 'Men in tights' to name a few, but this is a serious subject! Right?

2

HELP! I NEED SOMEBODY

"In addition to physical treatment, allowing patients time to talk and to discuss their fears and concerns is essential."

—Kelly Nickson,
Lymphoedema Clinical Nurse Specialist

Lymphoedema *is* a serious subject. Especially when newly diagnosed and you don't know what to do, how to adapt, how to treat it and where to go for help. In my case, the first six months were scary and left me feeling isolated, without much in the way of solutions, or even guidance as to how to deal with lymphoedema.

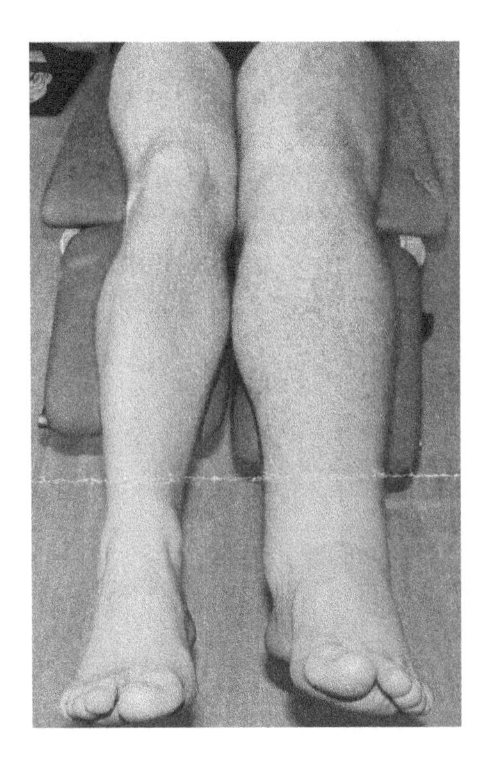

Matt's lower limb lymphoedema – November 2011

It's hard *not* to jump onto Google and become instantly terrified by the shocking, and in some cases, unimaginable images of extreme limb swelling. Could that be the future me? I needed to find someone to help me and fast! Horrifying thoughts ran through my mind of my leg increasing to the size of my waist, as seen in the images on Google. Since then, if I need to investigate a health-related issue, I only visit the official NHS UK website *www.nhs.uk* and use the search field. For example, if you type cellulitis into the NHS search field, you will find information, images and advice on when to call your GP, 111 or 999, which is very important if you suspect you have cellulitis. Such is the significance of cellulitis in lymphoedema, I have dedicated a chapter to this painful subject further into the book.

The first six months of living with lymphoedema really started to affect my mental wellbeing and personality. I have always been self-confident and stood tall, a happy and outgoing individual. Many people have told me over the years that I have a presence when I walk into a room, that I create a good impression and I am memorable, for all the right reasons, I might add. At this time of my life however, I was far from this person. I was desperately unhappy. At first, we blamed the quantity of drugs in my system, including morphine, for my moods and negativity. At its peak, my left leg was 56% bigger in volume than my right leg. I couldn't fit into any of my trousers and was unable to buy anything off the shelf that wasn't skin-tight (not a good look with lymphoedema) and my self-esteem and morale were plummeting rapidly. This was the closest that I had come to having depression.

So, I had to pick myself up, get back to real life and focus on my new business, which was launched just six months prior to me getting cellulitis and then lymphoedema. To stay professional and positive in front of the team, shield my physical discomfort, abnormal limb size and unusual clumsiness that my leg had created, was an unprecedented challenge for me. The stiff upper lip, carry on, "I'm fine!" barrier that I was putting up, possibly worked in the professional environment, but didn't fool those who knew me well.

Me - showing weakness and vulnerability - NEVER! In truth, I wasn't really coping at all well with the new challenges that lymphoedema had presented me, both physically and mentally. News Flash Hazledine! If I had acknowledged that I was struggling during this time and asked for help, I am confident that I would have received it from all quarters. But I didn't! I tried to carry on as normal, things to do, places to go, people to see. My attitude at the time was *"Men don't talk. That's a weakness. Don't show anyone a weakness, only strengths. Weaknesses are taken advantage of."* Ha! If my 50-year-old self, having lived with lymphoedema for 10 years, could talk to my 40-year-old self, the advice would be to seek help, talk to someone, perhaps a professional. You are not an island.

At this point, I would like to acknowledge and say thank you to my business partner at the time, Ian Painter and my wonderful team for carrying on without me and for their support and understanding during this period. It's bizarre looking back. I am naturally a problem solver, but during this time, I couldn't see a way to solve any of the problems that faced me as a result of having lymphoedema.

So, how did I manage to turn my life around? I am indebted to my wife and best friend, Victoria, or Vicki as she is known by all. Seeing me deteriorate like this prompted action and she started searching online to find help for people with lymphoedema. She visited forums, researched websites and had several phone conversations with various people in the sector. After two days of searching, Vicki spoke with a very helpful lady in Scotland and was told that the nearest lymphoedema clinic was based at The Hospice in the Weald, 10 minutes' drive from our home. Perfect! At last, a glimmer of hope, which transpired to be so vital in turning my life around and getting back on track.

During the first telephone conversation with one of their lymphoedema specialists, Kelly Nickson, Vicki was given a brief summary of their service, told to speak to our GP and ask for a referral to the hospice. Kelly explained that they would provide me with the much-needed treatment and ongoing care for lymphoedema. It was then that we heard the immortal words that we will never forget, *"Once we have Matt in our care, we won't let him go!"*. Wow, just typing that sentence has got my emotions going, I can tell you. It was just what we needed to hear at the time, and is also true to this day, as Kelly is supporting me with her contributions in my book.

On calling the GP for a referral to the Hospice in the Weald, the response was something like *"Oh, I thought that the hospice only dealt with cancer patients who had lymphoedema."* We had previously contacted our GP after leaving hospital, seeking help and guidance, which at that point was sadly missing. Time had marched on and it transpired that the help *was* actually there when I needed it the most, but neither we nor our GP knew about it. In 2016, the hospice disbanded the lymphoedema service to non-cancer outpatients and their operation was moved, coincidentally perhaps, to our local GP surgery. It is reassuring to know that any local people newly diagnosed with lymphoedema will be given the right help immediately, whilst those already with lymphoedema will receive the ongoing care they need.

I am so pleased to introduce you to Kelly Nickson who, although truly amazing, won't mind me saying that she isn't dissimilar to the majority of lymphoedema specialists and therapists I have met over the years, because they are all wonderful people. If you don't have a therapist, put that to the very top of your action list, but not until you have read Chapter 5 'Finding the right kind of therapist.'

At the end of November 2011, I had my first appointment with Kelly and her colleagues at the Hospice in the Weald and I remember feeling incredibly emotional. It surprised me when I spoke to Kelly recently that she still remembers that meeting to this day and she is happy to share her recollection. She was responsible for my treatment plan and quickly became a friend that I shared my concerns and emotions with, for which I am truly grateful. So, to give you a break from me for a while, I have the pleasure of introducing you to Kelly Nickson.

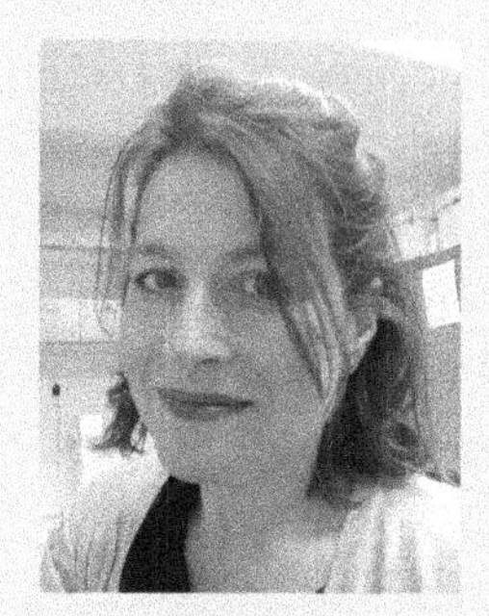

Kelly Nickson
Lymphoedema Clinical Nurse Specialist

I first met Matt and Vicki following his referral to the Lymphoedema clinic in 2011. Matt explained that he had been previously healthy, had a young family and enjoyed an active lifestyle, played sports, and took pride in his appearance. However, he explained that he no longer felt that he matched that description. He described feeling lost and unable to enjoy the same life that he had prior to developing lymphoedema which he attributed to a lack of available information and support after his diagnosis.

It was difficult for Matt to feel in control of his swelling without support, information and access to the correct aids to help him such as appropriate compression garments and self-care information. Working in the financial services profession Matt was used to wearing smart clothing and business attire; he described finding clothes and shoes to fit him in which he felt comfortable very difficult which is a common problem for people with lymphoedema. Matt was keen to seek help, advice and support and we were able to provide treatment for him.

During the time that Matt attended the clinic he tried a variety of treatments and strategies to improve his swelling including decongestive therapy, custom made flat knit garments and pneumatic compression as well as Kinesiology taping. Regular appointments to monitor his progress, assess his limb condition and obtain measurements for baseline comparison were important in enabling Matt to feel a degree of control over his swelling and to begin to understand what was most and least helpful to him. In addition to physical treatment allowing patients time to talk and to discuss their fears and concerns is essential. Matt has since undergone surgical options to achieve longer term management.

During the time that Matt was a patient at the clinic he presented at the Hospice AGM and was able to describe the experience of living with lymphoedema and the difficulty in finding treatment and support appropriate to his needs very eloquently. This was particularly important in an environment usually associated with cancer treatment and helped inform about the importance of access to care for people with all types of lymphoedema.

Having the opportunity to care for Matt in the first few years following his diagnosis highlighted to me the importance of timely and appropriate access to care as well as ensuring that patients and their families know that although their needs, both physical and psychological, will likely change over time, and that enabling self-management is an essential component of any treatment plan, specialist help and support will be there for them when they require it.

I would like to take this opportunity to sincerely thank Kelly Nickson and the team of therapists from Hospice in the Weald. They helped me at such a despairing time of my life and took such superb care of me for many years thereafter. Kelly helped me to climb out of the unfamiliar deep and dark hole that I found myself in.

After a few years of excellent specialist care, I was in a much better place physically and mentally. So much so as Kelly mentions, I was invited to present at the Hospice in the Weald Annual General Meeting in 2015. The purpose of my presentation was to explain to a room of around 50-60 influential people, the importance of their lymphoedema service to patients like me. I understood that the Board was reviewing the viability of continuing to provide this service to outpatients. It was a pleasure to represent their lymphoedema patients and to voice heartfelt thanks and appreciation to the lymphoedema team.

Kelly joins us again in Chapter 11 to provide important information and guidance regarding skin care.

So, who would I contact now if newly diagnosed and in need of finding a lymphoedema therapist? That is so much easier to answer now, as I would contact either or both The Lymphoedema Support Network (LSN) and The British Lymphology Society (BLS). Both organisations have a database of qualified therapists based in the UK and they can quickly sign-post you to those nearest to you. As I have previously mentioned, it is likely that you will first require a referral from your GP to see a therapist, but there is no harm in contacting the clinic to find out about their service in advance. Some therapists provide a private practice.

In my experience, it pays to understand your lymphoedema and the help that is available to you, which can only strengthen your case to be referred to the appropriate therapist for you. In my view, it is advisable to get into the system as soon as possible, as the swelling may worsen if you don't get the right care. I do not believe my leg was 56% bigger than the other leg when I left hospital. Had I got the expert help I needed sooner, I am confident that the swelling in my leg would not have increased as significantly and so quickly.

Top Tip #1: If diagnosed with lymphoedema, get a referral from your GP to a qualified therapist as soon as possible.

In the meantime, as I have alluded to already, knowledge is power and I would like to explain more about the actual condition/disease that is lymphoedema.

3

WHAT IS LYMPHOEDEMA?

"Continued research will lead to better investigations and treatments for all patients with lymphoedema in the future, but especially those with primary lymphoedema."

—Dr Kristiana Gordon MBBS,
CLT, MD(Res), FRCP

"Our understanding of secondary lymphoedema has had to be revised in recent years in light of a better understanding of the importance of the lymphatic system"

—Professor Vaughan Keeley PhD, FRCP

It's not often that I am asked about my leg by someone I don't really know, as I have become quite successful in hiding my lymphoedema. Now, I'm not normally one to draw attention to myself, well up until recently anyway. However, my answer to the few people who have asked me the question *"What's wrong with your leg?"* is very short and simple to avoid further in-depth and embarrassing discussion. *"I've got Lymphoedema. It's a swelling that develops when your lymphatic system is damaged or doesn't work properly"* followed swiftly by *"Did you see Match of the Day on Saturday..."* or *"Anyway, enough about me. How are you...?"*. This seems to work well enough for me. For those who know me well and are genuinely interested in why I've got a F'leg (fat leg), I am only too happy to discuss the condition with them. Sometimes it transpires that they know someone who has a swollen arm or leg but they were unaware it is called lymphoedema. I would suggest they pass on the details of the LSN, visit my new patient website *www.lymphoedemaunited.com* and buy a copy of this book.

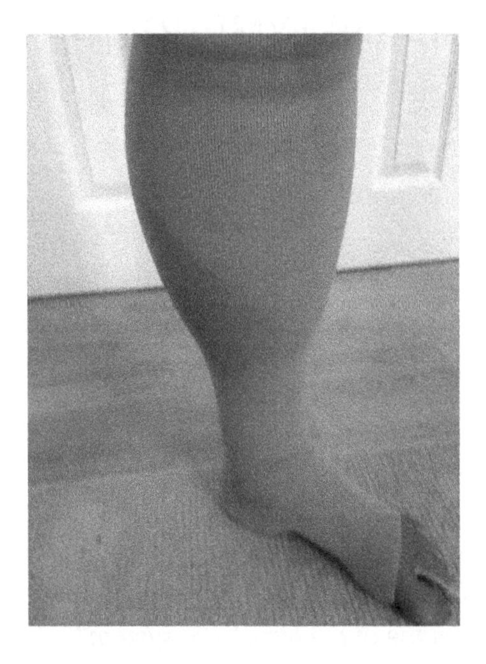

Matt's lower limb lymphoedema 2016 – before liposuction surgery

What is lymphoedema? In fact, there are two types of lymphoedema: primary and secondary. Primary is usually with you from birth and is typically associated with the failure or underdevelopment of the lymphatic system. Secondary is caused by external factors that prevent the lymphatic system from working properly, such as surgery, injury, trauma, infection, cancer and even obesity.

As I've already explained from the outset, I am not a medical expert in any capacity and have to be extremely careful what I say in this book. That is why I am privileged to introduce you to two esteemed healthcare professionals in the lymphoedema sector. First, my fabulously supportive consultant at St George's Hospital, Doctor Kristiana Gordon. I met Dr Gordon at my first NHS consultation appointment with Professor Peter Mortimer in 2012. Since then, she has been instrumental in improving my life with lymphoedema, especially in relation to applying for, and securing NHS funding for liposuction surgery, which has been life-changing for many reasons.

Dr Gordon has kindly agreed to explain primary lymphoedema.

Then, I am very grateful to Professor Vaughan Keeley, Consultant in Lymphoedema at Royal Derby Hospital, for explaining secondary lymphoedema. I have met Professor Keeley several times when attending his highly informative presentations, and when he has partaken in Q&A sessions as a member of a 'Panel of Experts.'

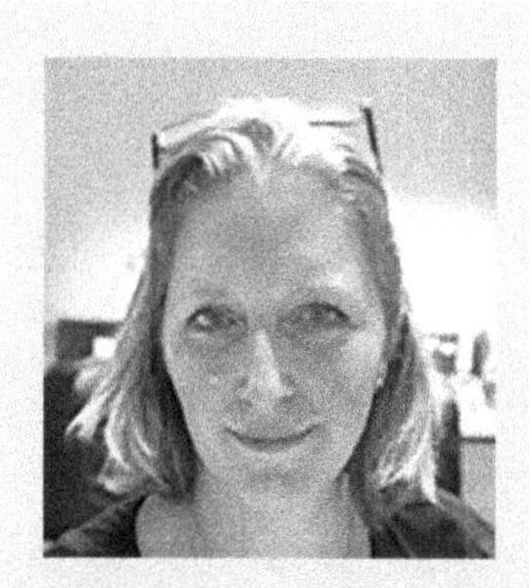

Dr Kristiana Gordon MBBS, CLT, MD(Res), FRCP
Consultant in Dermatology and Lymphovascular Medicine
St George's University Hospitals NHS Foundation Trust, London

I am a member of the lymphoedema team at St George's Hospital. I have supported Matt on his journey to secure a diagnosis and long-term management plan for his lymphoedema. I suspect Matt will agree that has been a journey filled with highs and occasional lows. I believe we have learnt a great deal from each other, both about an individual's response to lymphoedema treatment and the psychological impact this disease can inflict. I look forward to continuing to support Matt with managing his lymphoedema for many more years and am optimistic that the future of lymphoedema care will continue to develop and improve.

Introduction

Lymphoedema is the presence of chronic swelling (oedema) that occurs because of a failure of the lymphatic system to drain fluid from the spaces in-between the cells in our body. It may develop in someone with a previously healthy lymphatic system that has been damaged (for example, by cancer treatment) and this is called 'secondary lymphoedema.' This is the most common type of lymphoedema. 'Primary lymphoedema' occurs when someone is born with an abnormal lymphatic system. There are many different types of primary lymphoedema, and it should not be considered as one single condition.

What is Primary Lymphoedema?

Primary lymphoedema occurs as a result of a genetic fault causing the lymphatic system to fail to develop normally or to be adequately maintained. This causes abnormal drainage of lymphatic fluid resulting in swelling of the affected region (Figure 1). Someone with primary lymphoedema usually only has swelling of one or both lower limbs, but some rarer forms of primary lymphoedema may occur in association with other health problems (Connell et al 2010).

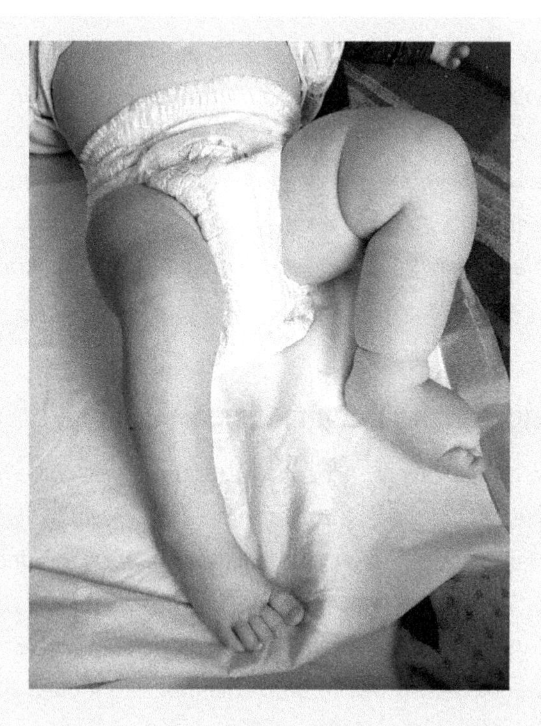

Figure 1: A boy born with lymphoedema of the left leg.

Primary lymphoedema may occur as an inherited condition from a parent who has passed on a genetic mutation, but frequently there is no known family history. Even though someone with primary lymphoedema will have the underlying genetic fault at birth, the swelling may not develop until later in life. Doctors don't really know how common primary lymphoedema is, but it has been estimated to affect at least 1 in every 1000 people (Moffatt CJ et al 2003).

Doctors have realised that primary lymphoedema is not one single disease, but the presenting feature of several distinct diseases, each with a different genetic mutation. Each type of primary lymphoedema is likely to have a different 'mechanism of disease', where a specific part of the lymphatic system fails to function normally. For example, some types of primary lymphoedema occur because of faulty valves within the lymphatic vessels (that are present to prevent backflow of lymph into the limb), and other types because of fluid absorption issues. It is important to understand the mechanism of lymphatic transport failure where possible, as doctors hope one day to be able to offer more targeted and effective treatments. In other words, we may be able to offer tailor-made treatment plans depending on the type of primary lymphoedema and the underlying gene mutation.

Diagnosing Primary Lymphoedema

Historically, primary lymphoedema was categorised into three groups based on the patient's age at the onset of their swelling: 'lymphoedema congenita' (swelling is present at birth), 'lymphoedema praecox' (pubertal onset) or 'lymphoedema tarda' (swelling onset after 35 years of age). Some doctors still use this rudimentary classification system, but it fails to take into account any health problems that might be associated with the lymphoedema.

It is now well established that the different types of primary lymphoedema vary in age of onset of the swelling, affected sites, possible associated health problems, inheritance patterns and the underlying genetic cause.

Mutations in several genes have been discovered to cause primary lymphoedema. Some, but not all, of these genes have been shown to play a role in lymphangiogenesis, the body's process of developing and maintaining a healthy lymphatic system. More than fifteen causal genes have now been discovered and can be tested for in specialist clinics, but these mutations are only present in a quarter of patients with primary lymphoedema. In other words, the underlying genetic cause of primary lymphoedema has been discovered in just 25% of cases. The other 75% will have an as-yet-undiscovered gene mutation. New gene mutations are continually being identified by lymphatic researchers. The discovery of these genes has influenced the diagnostic approach in the lymphoedema clinics, moving away from the age-based classification system to one that incorporates the different clinical signs and underlying genetic cause for each disease.

The clinical experience and research from the Primary Lymphoedema Clinic at St George's Hospital led to the realisation that primary lymphoedema can broadly be divided into five different categories, and that several distinct diseases fall within these 5 categories. Causal gene mutations have been identified for many of the diseases within these five categories and a colour-coded classification pathway has been developed to guide medical teams on how to correctly diagnose primary lymphoedema. (For further information, visit www.lymphoedemaunited.com/meet-the-experts/dr-kristiana-gordon/)

The five categories of primary lymphoedema represented in the new classification pathway are:

1 *(blue section): Lymphoedema associated with other genetic syndromes, such as Noonan or Turner syndrome (where lymphoedema is not the main feature of the patient's other health problems).*

2 *(pink section): Lymphoedema associated with systemic (internal) lymphatic abnormalities like fluid around the heart or lungs (e.g. Hennekam syndrome).*

3 *(yellow section): Lymphoedema that may be associated with lymphatic malformations, vascular malformations or overgrowth problems.*

4 *(green section): Congenital lymphoedema (this means it present at birth or within a few months of life), but there is no internal involvement and the lymphoedema is the predominant problem (e.g. Milroy disease).*

5 *(purple section): Lymphoedema that occurs later in life, after 1 year of age, but there is no internal involvement and the lymphoedema is the predominant problem (e.g. Lymphoedema Distichiasis Syndrome).*

Making the correct diagnosis is extremely important as it will allow doctors to identify what other problems the patient might be at risk of developing, and allow them to screen for them. Possible other health problems could include varicose veins, heart valve problems, immune problems, or internal lymphatic abnormalities. It is important to realise these are specific to the subtype of primary lymphoedema and most patients are not at risk of significant problems.

The classification pathway has been implemented in several countries including Europe and the United States of America. The impact has been to allow doctors to advise patients on what they can expect to happen from their disease and how best to avoid and manage the complications.

Management of Primary Lymphoedema

Unfortunately, gene therapy treatment is not yet available for primary lymphoedema. Until such time as 'drug treatments' become available, primary lymphoedema can be managed by physical treatments that improve swelling and reduce the risk of complications (such as cellulitis infections). These treatments are designed to stimulate lymphatic flow through existing or collateral drainage routes, and the approach is essentially the same as for patients with secondary lymphoedema.

Treatment should be overseen by a lymphoedema therapist and will usually involve the use of compression garments and/or bandaging regimes, with or without manual lymphatic drainage massage. Regular exercise, skin care (including management of cellulitis), weight management, and self-care are vital components of lymphoedema management. Psychological support must not be forgotten, as living with chronic lymphoedema can be difficult for patients (and parents) to come to terms with.

Whilst surgical techniques have been used in a bid to improve lymphatic drainage in patients with secondary lymphoedema they are not yet proven to significantly benefit patients with primary lymphoedema, presumably as patients do not have an 'obstruction' within their lymphatic system, but instead a molecular/genetic abnormality that cannot be bypassed with an operation.

Conclusion

The lymphatic system has been largely ignored by medical and scientific communities until recently, leading to a lack of progress in the management of lymphoedema compared to other diseases. Fortunately, doctors and scientists are now engaged as a result of recent advances in lymphatic research. The new classification pathway helps doctors to offer appropriate genetic testing (assuming the underlying gene mistake is known for the type of primary lymphoedema), and to screen and treat for any health problems occasionally associated with the type of primary lymphoedema. Patients and families benefit hugely from receiving a formal diagnosis of their condition as it allows doctors to confidently predict their clinical prognosis. The development of diagnostic genetic tests and recent pharmaceutical drug trials provides additional encouragement that more can be offered. Continued research will lead to better investigations and treatments for all patients with lymphoedema in the future, but especially those with primary lymphoedema.

References are listed in Appendix IV

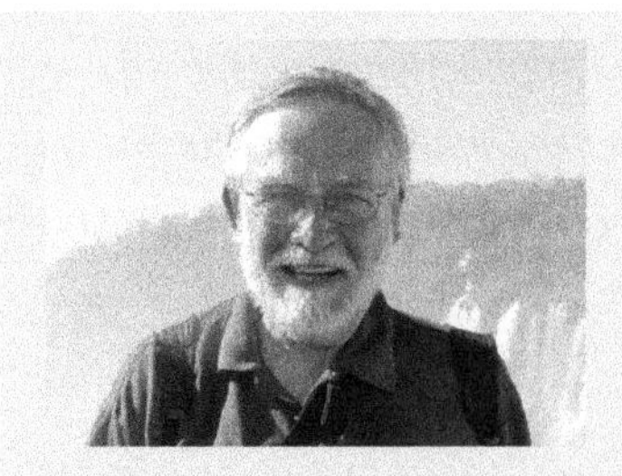

Professor Vaughan Keeley PhD, FRCP
Consultant in Lymphoedema, Derby Lymphoedema Service and Hon. Professor, University of Nottingham Medical School.

Introduction

I am a Medical Advisor to the LSN and met Matt at LSN conferences at which I have had the privilege to speak. I chair the LSN/BLS consensus group, which has drawn up guidelines on the management of cellulitis in Lymphoedema.

What is Secondary Lymphoedema?

Lymphoedema initially develops as swelling because of the build-up of fluid in the tissues (oedema) due to failure of the lymph system to drain it. Traditionally it has been divided into two types: primary lymphoedema (as described in the chapter by Kristiana Gordon) which is caused by a likely genetically determined problem with the development or maintenance of the lymphatic system, and secondary lymphoedema, which is usually thought of as damage to an otherwise normal lymphatic system by some external factor, such as surgery, radiotherapy and infection. Secondary lymphoedema has, therefore, often been considered to be largely due to cancer treatment in temperate climates and due to the parasitic infection, filariasis, in tropical climates.

However, our understanding of secondary lymphoedema has had to be revised in recent years in light of a better understanding of the importance of the lymphatic system in draining all excess fluid from the tissues and therefore being a key component in all types of chronic oedema. Chronic oedema will only occur if the lymphatic system fails to drain all the excess fluid from the tissues.

The term chronic oedema was defined to cover the wide range of chronic swelling seen in clinical settings, which previously had not been considered to be due to lymphoedema. For example, this would include chronic swelling due to venous disease, obesity, immobility, and chronic heart failure. In each of these conditions, swelling only occurs when the lymphatic system fails to keep up with the drainage of extra fluid arriving in the tissues from the blood capillaries. In some of these types of chronic swelling such as in venous disease there is a high flow of fluid into the tissues from the blood capillaries and if the lymphatic system is unable to drain it all away then swelling develops. In conventional lymphoedema, the lymphatic system is damaged and is therefore unable to drain enough fluid away even if there is not an excess arriving from the capillaries.

Therefore, increasingly, we are beginning to recognise all these types of chronic oedema to be due to a failure of the lymphatic system and therefore could be considered to be secondary lymphoedema.

In lymphoedema clinics, we see many people with chronic swelling e.g. of the legs, particularly in the elderly where the cause is due to a number of different factors. These include immobility perhaps due to arthritis or neurological conditions, obesity, venous disease such as varicose veins and sometimes heart failure. In addition, they may be taking medication, which can contribute to the swelling. Therefore, assessing which factors may be relevant in an individual patient is important in determining the best treatment for them.

Relatively little research on these different types of lymphoedema has been carried out in the past but, fortunately, there are more groups studying lymphoedema now and hopefully this will improve our understanding of the conditions.

Most of the research which has been carried out to date on secondary lymphoedema has focused on cancer treatment related lymphoedema but there have been small studies on other types such as that related to obesity and neurological conditions such as Multiple Sclerosis.

In this chapter, I will describe something of our current understanding of cancer-related lymphoedema and that related to obesity.

Cancer treatment-related lymphoedema:

Most of the research has been carried out on breast cancer-related lymphoedema but lymphoedema may also arise as a result of treatments for gynaecological cancer, prostate cancer, melanoma and head and neck cancers amongst others.

There is still a lot we do not know about why some women get lymphoedema of the arm after breast cancer treatment and others do not. There is increasing evidence of a possible genetic predisposition to developing secondary lymphoedema but this has not been fully identified as yet.

We also do not understand why it may take months or even years before the lymphoedema develops after breast cancer treatment and the simple model of damage to the lymphatic system arising from lymph-node removal in the armpit or radiotherapy treatment does not explain the pattern which we see.

We know that a number of factors may predispose to the development of breast cancer lymphoedema of the arm such as the woman's weight and the type of surgery and even some of the cancer treatments used such as taxane chemotherapy may increase the risk of developing it.

One of the current concepts is to try to identify those who are likely to develop lymphoedema of the arm following treatment so that we can intervene early in the hope of either reducing the severity of the problem or preventing it from developing altogether. Although research has identified certain risk factors, such that it may be possible to identify women who are more likely to develop lymphoedema, at present no particular intervention has been identified which is proven to prevent it from happening. Nevertheless, there may be some significant benefit from the early detection and treatment of mild lymphoedema, as it may reduce the risk of it increasing in severity over time. Some of the research evidence is encouraging in this area and from our own clinical experience, since we have been working closely with our local breast cancer unit and treating women with very mild lymphoedema promptly, we haven't seen as many women with more severe arm swelling as we used to some years ago.

Obesity and lymphoedema

There are a growing number of people presenting to lymphoedema clinics with lymphoedema predominantly of the legs due to weight problems.

We know that obesity has an impact on the venous circulation causing high venous pressure in the legs and also impairs lymphatic drainage. It is largely by these mechanisms that lymphoedema develops in this group. However, associated problems such as type II diabetes, obstructive sleep apnoea and reduced mobility may contribute.

We are also aware that obesity is a risk factor for developing cancer-related lymphoedema including that for breast cancer and that it is a risk factor for developing cellulitis in anyone with lymphoedema.

On the positive side, we are seeing evidence of improvement in the lymphoedema with sustained weight loss in many patients and in some to the point where it no longer requires any compression treatment. Although this is very encouraging, it is recognised that for many people, sustained weight loss is difficult to achieve.

Conclusions

The term secondary lymphoedema can be considered to cover a wide range of different conditions, which were previously not necessarily considered to be lymphoedema. It is far more common than primary lymphoedema. The causes in an individual patient may be quite complex and, therefore, a detailed assessment and, where appropriate, treatment of contributory factors such as heart failure and weight problems is helpful in achieving the best outcomes.

Pitting and Non-Pitting Oedema

During my consultation appointments at St George's Hospital, Dr Gordon would examine my leg and do a pitting test on my calf and thigh. Interestingly, I usually had pitting in my calf and non-pitting in my thigh. I have never asked her what the difference is between the two. So, while I had the opportunity, I asked Professor Keeley to provide a definition of Pitting and Non-Pitting oedema. His response was as follows:

Pitting oedema is oedema where the "pitting test" is positive. The pitting test involves pressing the skin firmly for at least 10 seconds in the area of swelling and seeing if a depression is left behind on removal of the pressure. If there is a depression, this is a positive test and is described as pitting oedema. If there is no depression then the test is negative. The interpretation of a negative test is slightly more complex - it could be negative if there is no oedema e.g. the swelling/enlargement is due to fat deposition or something else.

The term "non-pitting oedema" is best reserved to describe oedema which was previously pitting and has become non-pitting because of the inflammatory process which occurs in lymphoedema, which leads to a build up of fat and fibrosis in the tissues. Because the fluid element of the lymphoedema is minimal in this situation and the swollen tissue is predominantly composed of fat and fibrosis, it does not "pit" on pressure and so is described as "non-pitting oedema".

Thank you to both Dr Gordon and Professor Keeley for their time and thorough explanation.

What caused my lymphoedema?

In a clinic letter from Professor Mortimer in 2012, he wrote *"Your lymph gland biopsy shows quite marked fibrosis within the lymph gland which in my view confirms the diagnosis of ilioinguinal nodal sclerosis but does not tell us a reason." "What is certain is that it was the surgical intervention to his left groin that has really caused the obstruction and the severity of the lymphoedema he has today."*

Prior to the first episode of cellulitis in 2011, I'd had a bad fall carrying an oak table downstairs in my office. The significant bruising caused by the fall, combined with an open blister from wearing my new golf shoes and previous surgery to remove my inguinal lymph nodes, created the perfect storm to trigger my lymphoedema.

Do I have primary or secondary lymphoedema?

This is a discussion that Professor Mortimer and I have had a few times over the years. He is of the opinion that this perfect storm triggered my dormant primary lymphoedema. The only reason I really care which type it is, is to find out whether or not it is hereditary. Could my daughters have it?

I share this part of my story in case you can relate to some of my early warning signs that I perhaps should have paid more attention to at the time. If you, or someone you know experiences any of these symptoms, and that's what they are, symptoms, then I would suggest that you speak to your GP as soon as possible.

I had experienced a puffy ankle during late teenage years and thought nothing of it. At the age of 16, I swapped my entrepreneurial car cleaning round to work as a weekend shop assistant in our local hardware store. This involved being on my feet from 8.30am to 6pm every Saturday and 8.30am to 1.30pm every Sunday. I loved that job, but I do remember an unusually hot summer when, by the end of the day, my ankles, more so my left, were noticeably puffy. But, as a teenager, I was more interested in going home, eating dinner, getting changed to go back out and meet my friends for either a game of football, snooker, tennis, badminton, or golf depending on the weather and how much sunlight was left. I didn't think it important to mention my puffy ankle to my parents as it soon went down again to normal size. Anyway, my mind was on other things as it was exam year at school, so revising and then hanging out with my mates was more important.

In my 20s and 30s, I would experience puffy ankles, especially my left one, as a result of flights abroad, but again thought nothing of it. I am sharing this with you as these are signs of primary lymphoedema, so I have been subsequently told.

A few years prior to the cellulitis attack, at the age of 36, I had an urgent appointment with my GP complaining of a severe pain in the left hand-side of my groin area, me not my GP. So much so, I found it impossible to stand up straight. After his initial examination and a failed (and rather painful) manipulation attempt, he made a telephone call and told me to go straight to the hospital, where they were expecting me within the hour. His diagnosis was a possible strangulated hernia, which is fairly serious apparently and requires urgent medical treatment.

On arrival at the A&E Department on a wintry January Friday afternoon, I gave my personal details to the receptionist and was taken straight to a bed in a ward and told to get into a gown. A nurse did my observations, or 'obs' as it's called in the trade. ('obs' being blood pressure, pulse and temperature.)

I recall a doctor examining me and trying to manipulate my hernia back into place, again without success. Shortly after that attempt, a surgeon in his blue scrubs joined us and examined the area of pain. He too attempted to manipulate my 'hernia' back into position, again without success. He announced that I was to have emergency surgery and for the nurses to get me ready and sent down to theatre. It was only a couple of hours ago that I was at my local GP surgery, it all happened so fast.

I phoned my then girlfriend, Vicki, who was at work in London, telling her not to worry before calmly explaining that I was on my way to theatre for surgery to sort out a strangulated hernia. I didn't have long, but enough time to say *"all will be fine, I love you and I'll see you later on"*. Within one hour of hobbling bent over into A&E, I was taken down to theatre.

It turned out that it wasn't a strangulated hernia after all. The surgeon told me that the pain was caused by enlarged lymph nodes, which he had removed and sent off for biopsy to see if they were cancerous. Then he left. It was around 5pm on a Friday afternoon and although I was feeling typically groggy from the anaesthetic, hearing the words *"to see if they are cancerous"* instantly got my attention. It was like an over-sized bucket of ice-cold water being thrown over my face.

Then came the agonising and worrying wait. Thankfully, the results of the biopsy were negative and there weren't any signs of cancer which was, of course, a massive relief. However, I think I can safely say that oddly, this was the calm before the storm that was soon to follow. As this surgery had been considered an emergency for a strangulated hernia, the surgeon had made the decision to remove the problematic lymph nodes, clearly without any conversation about possible subsequent repercussions. He made his decision during surgery, no doubt with good intention, with the protection that I had signed the appropriate waiver forms.

Years later, in his letter to me dated 29 October 2012, Professor Mortimer wrote *"What is certain is that it was the surgical intervention to his left groin that has really caused the obstruction and the severity of the lymphoedema he has today."*

Moving on to September 2010, we took a well needed two-week family holiday to Spain. This turned out to be the last time that both my legs would be tanned. The last time that I would be playing merrily around the swimming pool and on the beach with my youngest daughter, without an ugly 'here I am' compression stocking on my left leg. During the second week, my left heel became very painful to walk on. The skin had become cracked and my ankle puffy. I put it down to a combination of the chlorine in the pool, with the salt of the sea, with the heat and maybe the sand drying out the skin. It became so very painful and difficult to walk, that I bought some new sliders with thick cushioned soles, which eased the discomfort somewhat. Can you see where this is heading? I certainly didn't!

In June 2011, I fell down some stairs in our office, whilst carrying a very heavy oak table with my business partner. This fall caused some impressively multi-coloured bruising on my derrière. Around the same time, I also got a blister on the little toe of my left foot, wearing some brand-new golf shoes that I'd received as a 40th birthday present.

So, can you see where this is going now? Yes, spot on! A week or so later, on the day before Father's Day in June 2011, I fell poorly very quickly, had cellulitis which then resulted in lymphoedema, as previously mentioned.

The moral of the story is to holiday in Portugal, get a lighter table and play golf in trusted old shoes.

Therefore, my story has resulted in much deliberation to establish whether I had primary or secondary lymphoedema. Professor Mortimer is convinced I had dormant primary lymphoedema and the trigger was the cellulitis infection. Perhaps the bugs got in during my Spanish holiday? Not the best souvenir that I've brought back, that's for sure. I think, and I'm sure I'm in denial, that it was secondary lymphoedema caused by surgery, injury and infection. However, as I have declared already, I'm no expert and who am I to argue with Professor Peter Mortimer?

In my opinion, it is worthwhile asking your parents and grandparents if they have or had any swollen or puffy limbs, as it might be lymphoedema and therefore, it might be hereditary. You can then research the condition as you may be at risk of getting it in future. There are steps you can take to try and reduce or prevent lymphoedema, some of which are covered in this book.

Condition or Disease?

In my 10 years' experience of talking about lymphoedema with various UK medical experts and organisations (many of whom are in my book), lymphoedema is more frequently referred to as a chronic condition and not a disease. This is consistent with my research of many websites and books too, including the NHS definition: *"Lymphoedema is a long-term (chronic) condition that causes swelling in the body's tissues. It can affect any part of the body, but usually develops in the arms or legs. It develops when the lymphatic system does not work properly."*

During an email conversation with William Repicci, President & CEO of Lymphatic Education & Research Network (LE&RN) based in New York, I referred to lymphoedema as a condition. His very lengthy response included some extremely strong views about my referencing. I will summarise this. In the USA, Lymphedema (LE) is referred to as a disease and never a condition by LE&RN, to raise the significance in the eyes of those with lymphedema and the public in general. It is felt that the term 'condition' is used by the medical profession to soften the impact for the patients, so it's not considered on the same par as cancer or diabetes. As one LE&RN patient says *"You can live with a condition. We cure diseases. I want a cure"*. It is William's view that for LE&RN to drive a global effort for a cure, LE needs to be communicated as a disease to elevate its importance alongside other more well-known diseases.

I enjoyed the email interaction with William and am very respectful of his opinion and powerful argument that lymphedema/lymphoedema/LE should be referred to only as a disease and not a condition. However, I did take the opportunity to share my own personal view, which is that I don't like to refer to *my* lymphoedema as a disease, as I associate disease with death.

Another reason for calling it a condition may have something to do with the great British stiff upper lip and 'Carry On' attitude. I have never said to friends or family, that I have a disease called lymphoedema. I do refer to it as a lifelong condition and try to play it down, but that's just me. So, in summary, I guess William makes a very valid point.

4

HOW COMMON IS CHRONIC OEDEMA?

"Lymphoedema affects approximately 250 million people worldwide. The proportion of individuals affected by Chronic Oedema is likely to be much higher than we currently believe."

—Professor Christine J. Moffatt CBE

Professor Vaughan Keeley mentioned chronic oedema in his chapter. Let's find out more about it. Chronic oedema is defined as a persistent swelling in soft tissue which has been present for more than three months and which does not completely reduce overnight or with elevation. This includes lymphoedema. Chronic oedema is most common due to problems with the venous and lymphatic systems and it is a progressive and debilitating condition that requires long-term management.

It is reported that, as the ageing population increases, the number of people with chronic oedema will increase over the coming years. Obesity will also contribute to an increase in the number of people with chronic oedema, which is why lymphoedema experts and medical professionals consistently advocate healthy lifestyle choices including movement and healthy eating.

I can only recall knowing one person with chronic oedema or lymphoedema. I say know, but just as a passing 'hello' and brief pleasantries. I don't have any friends or family members with the condition. After I was diagnosed, I had no one to call on who truly understood what it's like living with lymphoedema. That felt quite lonely and isolating.

However, based on the latest estimates, the British Lymphology Society (BLS) state on their website that *"there are estimated to be almost 450,000 people in the UK with lymphoedema"*. Where are these people?

Lymphatic Education & Research Network (LE&RN) report that *"The World Health Organization estimates that over 250 million people worldwide have secondary lymphedema, while primary lymphedema affects an additional 1 in 300 live births. Nearly 1.4 billion people in 73 countries are threatened by lymphatic filariasis, commonly known as elephantiasis. Over 120 million people are currently infected, with 40 million disfigured and incapacitated by the disease".*

Therefore, why didn't I know anyone else with the disease at that time? The first time I properly met other people with lymphoedema who understood the condition, was at the Lymphoedema Support Network (LSN) Annual General Meeting in London in 2015. In a room full of around 100 people, it was notable there were only three men with lymphoedema, including myself. That said a lot to me at the time and I have more to say on this later.

So, how common is chronic oedema? I first met Professor Christine Moffatt at a BLS conference when I was a trustee of the LSN. She provided a very informative and comprehensive presentation. Based on my first impression, she is the human encyclopaedia on chronic oedema and very delightful with it. We spoke recently during lockdown via video call and Professor Moffatt was very generous with her time and encouraging of my projects. In what is considered quite a niche disease, I asked her how common is chronic oedema? The answer below is kindly provided jointly by Professor Moffatt and Martina Sykorova.

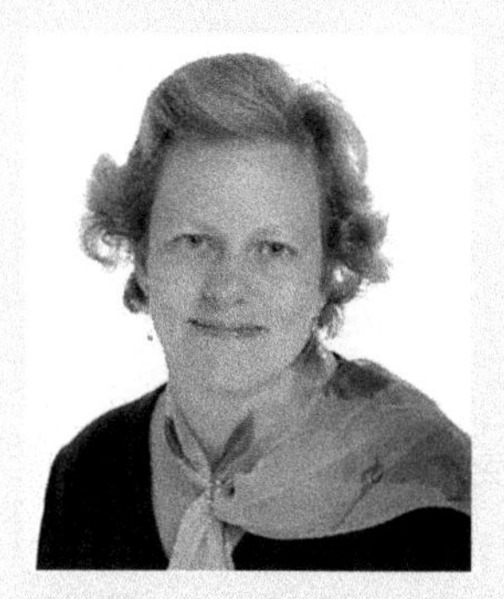

Professor Christine J. Moffatt CBE
Nottingham University Hospital and Emeritus Professor University of Nottingham

Professor Moffatt is a nurse by background and has worked in the field of wound care and lymphoedema for three decades including with Peter Mortimer at St. George's Hospital for 20 years. She is a clinician and is particularly interested in showing how many people are affected with the condition and the impact is has on patients' lives.

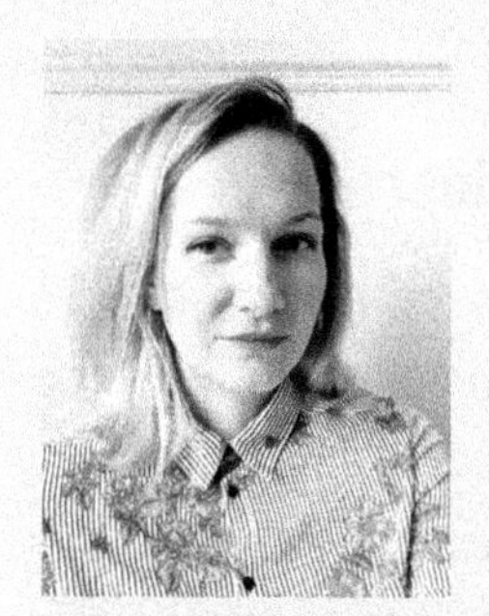

Martina Sykorova Bc., Mgr., MA, MRes
PhD Researcher, University of Nottingham

Martina has a background in public health and has been researching chronic oedema since 2014. Martina's current research is looking into the evaluation of a pathway for patients with chronic oedema and wet legs treated in the community.

What do the words Lymphoedema or Chronic Oedema mean?

Chronic oedema is defined as a swelling that has been present for more than three months and involves more than one body area[1]. Chronic oedema affects all parts of the body, people of all ages, and both sexes. The term 'chronic oedema' is an umbrella term which includes various types of long-term swelling, and Primary and Secondary Lymphoedema. There is not one cause of Chronic Oedema, instead people can develop Chronic Oedema due to several reasons such as venous disease, lymphatic disease, immobility or systemic disease. The word Chronic Oedema is therefore not a diagnosis, but a public health term used to describe the many different types of the condition. Lymphoedema occurs due to the damage of the lymphatic system which can be primary (from birth) or secondary (for example due to cancer or an infection such as Lymphatic Filariasis). Lymphoedema is a lifelong condition requiring a lifelong treatment. It is important that all patients receive a clinical assessment that can provide the correct diagnosis.

How common is Chronic Oedema worldwide?

Lymphoedema affects approximately 250 million people worldwide[2], of those 120 million people are affected by a neglected tropical disease Lymphatic Filariasis, a type of lymphoedema caused by a mosquito bite. Lymphatic Filariasis occurs mainly in India and Africa and causes mainly genital lymphoedema in men (25 million) and elephantiasis of the leg in women mostly (15 million)[3]. In fact we do not know how many people are affected by Chronic Oedema in the world because of the many different conditions associated with it.

How common is Chronic Oedema in the UK?

Currently we do not know the exact number of individuals living with Chronic Oedema in the UK. Lymphoedema has historically been linked to having cancer, which is likely to be the cause in only around a third of people. Previous research studies show that Chronic Oedema occurs in 1.33[4]-3.99[5] individuals in 1,000 population in various parts of England. This means that we can estimate that there are between 76,000 and 227,000 people living with Lymphoedema in England[6] and between 7,000 and 21,000 in Scotland[7]. It is estimated that 2,274 individuals are affected by lymphoedema in Northern Ireland[8] although this number was calculated using older estimates and is likely to be at least three-times higher. In Wales it is estimated that Lymphoedema occurs in 6.64 in 1000 people which equals to 20,935 individuals living with Lymphoedema in the year 2020 - 2021[9]. The English, Scottish and Northern Irish are based on two studies published in 2003 and 2012 (1.33 and 3.99 in 1,000 people). If we use the most up-to-date Welsh estimates (6.64 in 1000 people) and apply them to the rest of the UK the prevalence of Lymphoedema would equate to 443,530 (figure 1). However, it is important to note that the approximate numbers are likely to be an under-estimate of the true numbers because some individuals with Chronic Oedema are not diagnosed and therefore unknown to the healthcare system.

	Population (2019)[10]	2003 London prevalence estimate (1.33 per 1000)	2012 Derby prevalence estimate (3.99 per 1000)	2021 Welsh prevalence estimate (6.64 per 1000)
England	56,286,961	74,862	224,585	373,745
Scotland	5,463,300	7,266	21,799	36,276
Wales	3,152,879	4,193	12,580	20,935
Northern Ireland	1,893,667	2,519	7,555	12,574
UK TOTAL	66,796,807	88,840	266,519	443,530

Figure 1: Lymphoedema prevalence estimates in the UK

In the UK Chronic Oedema affects a large proportion of patients that are being treated in their own homes by community nurses. It is important to note that patients on a community nursing caseload tend to be older than the general population, present with other chronic conditions and experience issues with their mobility. A recent study conducted in Leicester and Nottingham showed that almost 57% of patients who are treated in their own homes by community nurses suffer from Chronic Oedema[11]. Chronic Oedema is also common in hospital patients. A study conducted in a number of European hospitals showed that 38% of hospital patients presented with Chronic Oedema[12]. Similarly Chronic Oedema affects a large number of care home residents, however, there is a limited data available regarding this patient group. More research is needed to better understand the size and impact of Chronic Oedema on care home residents[13].

The chances of developing chronic oedema are closely associated with higher age and suffering from other long-term health conditions such as venous disease and cancer. The number of Chronic Oedema cases within a population increases significantly in individuals over 85, the number is three-times higher compared to those aged over 65[14] and seven-times higher compared to the general adult population[15]. Moreover, women are more likely to develop Chronic Oedema[16, 17].

Individuals who present with chronic oedema are at a higher risk of developing other conditions such as leg ulcers (in a 2016 study 40% of patients with Chronic Oedema also had a concurrent leg ulcer[18]) and cellulitis, a bacterial infection that affects deeper layers of the skin and can lead to serious complications if not treated early. It is estimated that 37% of people with Chronic Oedema will develop cellulitis during their lifetime[19]. Obesity is another factor that negatively influences patients with lymphoedema by increasing the risk of infection, being hospitalised and having a larger limb[20].

How common is Primary Lymphoedema?

Primary Lymphoedema is a rare condition that is caused by malformations to the lymphatic system which may be hereditary. Unlike Secondary Lymphoedema that accounts for over 90%[21, 22] of all Lymphoedema cases, it is not possible to prevent the development of Primary Lymphoedema[23]. It is estimated that Primary Lymphoedema affects 1 in 6,000[24] although a recent study conducted in two English areas showed that it affected 1 in 2,763 and 1 in 5,129[25]. Difficulties in the accuracy of diagnosis may mean that people have not been correctly classified as to whether they have Primary or Secondary Lymphoedema.

How common is Cancer-Related Lymphoedema?

Historically Secondary Lymphoedema has been linked to cancer or cancer treatment although cancer-related Lymphoedema only affects a minority of the overall cases. Secondary Lymphoedema can be associated with many other factors such as diabetes, lymphovenous disease, obesity and immobility[26]. Studies estimate that Secondary Lymphoedema affects 2 in 10 of breast cancer survivors[27], 5 in 10 with vulvar cancer survivors, and 3 in 10 with penile cancer survivors[28].

How common are wet legs?

'Wet legs' or 'lymphorrhea' occur in grossly oedematous legs, when the body cannot cope with the excess fluid. The skin breaks resulting in leakage of the excess fluid outside patient's legs[29]. Wet legs are a symptom of untreated or uncontrolled chronic oedema. Currently it is unknown how common the condition is within the UK. It is estimated that it accounts for 6% of all wound types on a community nursing caseload in eight UK areas[30], however, this number is likely to be an underestimate of the true problem because lymphorrhea can be confused for a leakage from a wound.

Conclusion

Although there is scientific evidence of how common Chronic Oedema is in specific parts of the UK or how common Lymphoedema is in certain patient groups such as breast cancer patients, the impact and spread of chronic oedema within the general population within the UK remains unknown. The proportion of individuals affected by Chronic Oedema is likely to be much higher than we currently believe.

References 1-30 are listed in Appendix IV

Thank you both for such a comprehensive and informative answer to my question.

5

FINDING THE RIGHT KIND OF THERAPIST

"Being under the care of a specialist practitioner who is both qualified and experienced in managing lymphoedema offers the best opportunity to ensure your lymphoedema is reduced as much as possible."

—Margaret Sneddon,
Chair, British Lymphology Society

Just to recap, in 2011, after a severe episode of cellulitis I was first diagnosed with lymphoedema. After a 13-night stay, I was discharged from hospital without any information, guidance or signposts on where to go for help. It was a daunting prospect. This condition had come on so quickly following such an excruciatingly painful infection. This little-known disease was with me and I needed expert advice and care. After several days of internet searching and numerous phone calls, we found a team of experienced lymphoedema therapists just a 10-minute drive away.

I appreciate now, that I am one of the lucky ones. Currently, there is a reducing number of qualified lymphoedema therapists in the UK. The clinics that do provide this service may not be so easily accessible for many people with this, often, debilitating condition.

Today, however, it's much easier to find a therapist online using Google search, or is it? I decided to find out. I typed "Lymphoedema therapist near me" into Google search and 14 red pins appeared in the Kent map, within a 30-minute drive from home. This is where further research is highly recommended, due to the search engine picking up the keyword 'therapist.' Clicking on each red pin in turn and visiting the relevant website, gave me more information about the services provided to enable me to make a shortlist. Out of the 14 listed, here are the results:

- 2 were hospitals
- 4 were GP surgeries, without any therapists featured on their websites. The irony is that one of them is my local GP, where I know for a fact the NHS West Kent Lymphoedema Clinic is based, including two therapists I've known for years. They provide the full complement of services: Multi-Layer Lymphoedema Bandaging (MLLB), Manual Lymphatic Drainage (MLD) and measure and arrange supply of compression garments, all on the NHS. Why don't they feature on the website, or have a website of their own? I will ask the question!
- 1 was a GP surgery that featured physiotherapy as one of their services
- 2 were beauty therapists providing beauty therapy, massage, reflexology, aromatherapy
- 1 was a clinic providing every kind of therapy except for lymphoedema, including: physiotherapy, osteopathy, sports massage, homeopathy, aromatherapy, reflexology and hypnotherapy

- 2 provided reflexology, both listing a therapy I hadn't heard of before called Reflexology Lymph Drainage (RLD) more on this in Chapter 14.
- 2 websites were for the same person - Clare Anvar MSc, who provides clinical therapies for lymphoedema, including Manual Lymphatic Drainage (MLD) and Kinesio Taping. She also provides intensive daily Decongestive Lymphatic Therapy (DLT), including Multi-Layer Lymphoedema Bandaging (MLLB). The price for MLD was £75 per hour. I have been to Clare several times for post-surgical treatment after liposuction and have to say that her service is excellent. I am pleased to say that Clare joins us in Chapter 14.

One of the important signs that reassured me that I would find a qualified and experienced therapist to treat my lymphoedema, was that two of the websites featured the logos of the British Lymphology Society (BLS) and the Lymphoedema Support Network (LSN). This means that the therapist is a member of these organisations and is listed on their Directory.

I would recommend that you check The BLS Member Service Directory when looking for a therapist *www.thebls.com/directory.* This enables members to declare what training they have undertaken and the dates of their MLD updates (usually recommended every two years). However, it is important to know that the BLS and the LSN are not regulatory bodies, so cannot 'approve' anyone.

It has also been suggested to me, to check that the healthcare professional is registered with the Nursing and Midwifery Council or Health Professional Council, who are the regulatory bodies and ensure that no one provides treatment beyond their scope of practice. Other therapists are likely to be registered with MLD^{UK}. Checking their website will show if they are trained to provide all aspects of lymphoedema therapy or only specific aspects *www.mlduk.org.uk/therapists*. More about MLD^{UK} in Chapter 14.

The BLS promotes professional standards in lymphoedema care and treatment. Their other aims are to benefit patients by improving the knowledge, expertise and skills of healthcare professionals treating them, and to produce and maintain a register of specialist centres in the UK and Ireland. I was first introduced to Margaret Sneddon, Chair, at a BLS conference in 2017, when I was a trustee of the LSN. I was very flattered that Margaret remembered me, when I contacted her back in February 2021, inviting her to contribute to this chapter. Margaret agreed that this is, indeed, a very important subject close to her heart and one of the focuses of the BLS. It is with great pleasure that I handover to Margaret, asking her how people with lymphoedema can be sure to find the right kind of qualified therapist to provide appropriate treatment, both initially with decongestion and ongoing management.

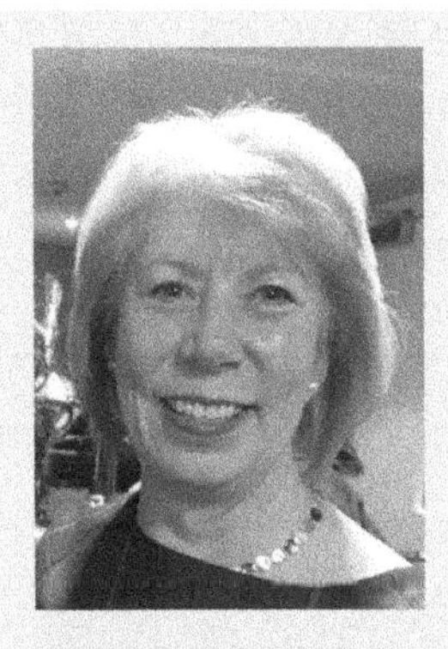

Margaret Sneddon
Chair, British Lymphology Society / Sen. Hon. Research Fellow (Former Head of Dept/Lead for lymphoedema education & research, University of Glasgow)

Introduction

Matt and I met briefly at a British Lymphology Society (BLS) conference a few years ago but had not really communicated until we were reintroduced fairly recently by Prof. Peter Mortimer, founder and Patron of the BLS. Peter and I have known each other for over 30 years through our shared interest in lymphoedema, education and involvement in the British

Lymphology Society and he knew I, and the BLS would be both interested and supportive of Matt's aspiration to develop a web-based resource for people with lymphoedema. There are many gaps in provision of care, support and knowledge in relation to lymphoedema and Matt had certainly identified with some of these through his own harrowing experiences. Filling these gaps needs a multidimensional approach and for all of us who are passionate about doing so to collaborate. I am delighted that Matt and the BLS are continuing discussions about how we can work together effectively and am honoured to be invited to contribute to this book.

You and your specialist practitioner

Once a diagnosis of lymphoedema has been established, being under the care of a specialist practitioner who is both qualified and experienced in managing lymphoedema offers the best opportunity to ensure your lymphoedema is reduced as much as possible, the reduction maintained, and any problems and complications avoided.

Healthcare professionals or therapists who have successfully completed recognised training as a specialist lymphoedema practitioner generally do so because they are passionate about lymphoedema and providing the best possible care for anyone referred to them. They are likely to ensure that they are familiar with new developments and products available for their patients by updating their knowledge and skills on a regular basis and attending conferences and meetings with other specialists in the field, such as the BLS annual conference. Many will be members of the British Lymphology Society (BLS), actively support the work of BLS and have their service included in the Service Directory. This is more than a listing as it clearly identifies the types of treatment offered, the training undertaken by practitioners and dates of any updates attended. Some small services are unable to offer all types of treatment but will recognise when something else would be helpful for you and advise or refer on to other specialists as required.

Engaging as an expert in your own lymphoedema

Your experience of lymphoedema and its impact on your life; treatment needs to be tailored to meet your specific needs. An experienced lymphoedema practitioner will recognise you as the expert in your own condition, even although initially you may feel angry and bewildered following diagnosis and very dependent on your specialist practitioner who holds all the knowledge. Over time, your relationship with your specialist practitioner will evolve as they help you understand more about lymphoedema and be able to recognise how your body responds to treatments and your own activities, enabling you to become more confident in the day-to-day management of your lymphoedema, minimising its impact on your life and being less dependent on health care professionals.

Getting to this stage of feeling in control of your lymphoedema, rather than lymphoedema controlling everything you do is easier if you and your practitioner work in partnership to achieve what is most important to you. For example, it may be more important to you to reduce discomfort, enable you to do certain things you enjoy or wear a more comfortable compression garment, than to see the size of the swelling go down a bit more. Sharing what is important to you and monitoring what makes your lymphoedema worse and what makes it better is really helpful in getting your treatment right and also in understanding the things that you can do help your lymphatic system work as well as possible.

Even if your practitioner is unable to provide all types of specialist treatment, they will recognise when they are needed and be able to advise and refer you to an appropriate practitioner. Compression garments are, of course, a key part of treatment and there are literally thousands of options in terms of strength, stiffness, fit, material, style and colour, most available on prescription. There are also many different aids for applying compression garments. It can be a bit of trial and error to get your best option and you should not be confined to garments from one company. Your specialist practitioner will be able to discuss alternatives and advise what is available on prescription or for personal purchase.

Engaging with practitioners who are not lymphoedema specialists

It is well recognised that there are too few lymphoedema specialists and that not everyone who has lymphoedema has access to any such specialist. Excellent care may also be provided by specialist health care professionals in relevant fields who have undertaken training in the management of lymphoedema for their specific patient group. Examples may include nurses, physiotherapists or occupational therapists specialising in breast cancer, burns or tissue viability. Such practitioners are very skilled but may have fewer opportunities to keep up-to-date with new products or treatments as someone dealing exclusively with lymphoedema. However, they will be able to consult with or refer to more specialist colleagues when required. So again, you should not feel you need to accept the first option offered and never be afraid to share concerns or ask if there are any alternatives.

Unfortunately, interest and pursuit of knowledge of lymphoedema depends on the individual professional and service. The British Lymphology Society now encourages non-specialist healthcare professionals (and others) to register as a Friend of BLS at no cost. This allows them to access free information, updates about lymphoedema and its treatment and links to resources by the BLS and other organisations, providing information and useful tips for both healthcare professionals and people with lymphoedema. It may be worth drawing this to the attention of the healthcare professionals responsible for your care in case they are unaware. If you feel your lymphoedema is not managed well, you can ask to be referred to a specialist.

For many people with lymphoedema the main professional healthcare support may be provided by the Primary Care Team, such as your general practitioner (GP), community or general practice nurse, all of whom have a care remit for patients with a wide variety of health problems. It may be that your lymphoedema has been caused, or contributed to, by conditions in which they have substantial experience. Although they cannot be expected to have specialist knowledge in every condition and may have very limited experience of lymphoedema management, they may play a key role in your long-term maintenance and support, especially once your condition and management is stable. Most will recognise their own limitations and seek out information to help them support you, be willing to listen to any concerns and questions, following these up with specialists colleagues if necessary. They may also be very happy to be given links to reputable sources of information such as the British Lymphology Society resources and register as a Friend of BLS to keep up-to-date.

Although it is not your role to educate professionals, having a good relationship and engaging with your GP or other professionals in the practice will undoubtedly enhance their understanding of the condition, your needs and how they can help. Even if you have access to a lymphoedema specialist, maintaining contact with your GP service is helpful. You have access to a wide range of professional help through your GP service, such as help in losing weight with the support of a dietician or referral to weight management groups, getting more active with the support of local fitness clubs and trainers. Make the most of whatever support is available to help you manage your lymphoedema and prevent any problems.

To find your nearest qualified lymphoedema therapist, please visit www.thebls.com/directory

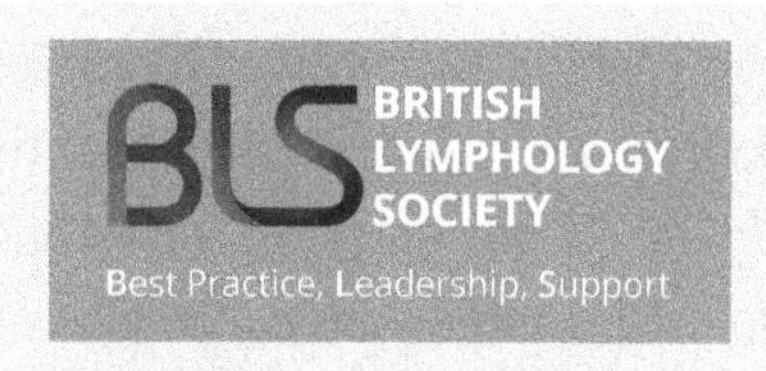

The British Lymphology Society

The British Lymphology Society (BLS) is a UK charitable incorporated organisation. Our underpinning purpose is to preserve and protect good health of people living with lymphoedema / chronic oedema. Lymphoedema occurs when the lymphatic drainage system fails; chronic oedema is indicative of failure of lymphatic drainage. Our charitable purpose uses both these interchangeable terms to emphasise the need to manage both the initial cause of the chronic oedema and the lymphatic failure concurrently.

In pursuit of our key purpose we strive for a reduction in the prevalence, severity and impact of lymphoedema by two main strategies:

1 Enhancing awareness, understanding, recognition and interest in lymphoedema

- We believe that healthcare professionals of all disciplines who know what lymphoedema is, what are the causes, contributory factors and early signs and symptoms, will be equipped to recognise who is at risk, provide advice on self-care to reduce the likelihood of developing lymphoedema and ensure prompt diagnosis and intervention should it develop. They will also be able to provide ongoing monitoring and support to help those living with lymphoedema, knowing when and how to either refer to, or consult with, a specialist lymphoedema practitioner.
- We believe in a need for wider public awareness of lymphoedema, how common it is and that most of us are at risk at some stage in our lives – to realise that lymphoedema is important.

We want everyone to take any swelling seriously, to know what they can do themselves and when to seek help. The support of Trisha Goddard, TV presenter, as our second Patron has been hugely helpful in being a very public face of our campaigning and capturing public attention for lymphoedema.

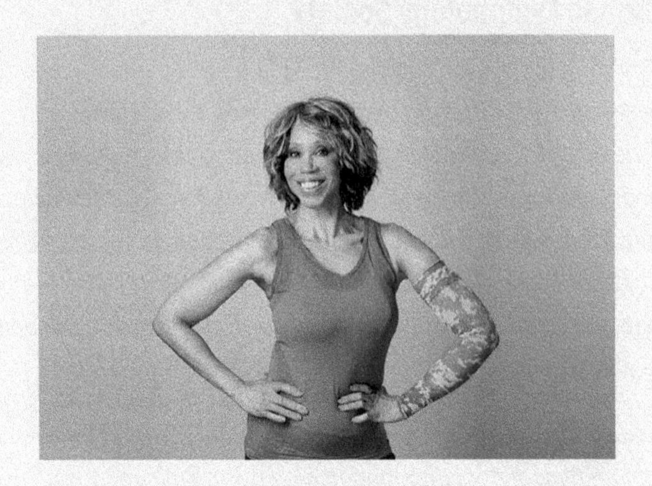

Trisha Goddard – Patron of the British Lymphology Society

2 Enhancing knowledge and skills in the diagnosis and management of lymphoedema

- We are passionate about promoting the best possible standards of care and treatment; our members support this through their contributions to BLS outputs, including the sharing of research, tools, strategies and resources to guide clinical practice, delivering presentations, writing for publications.
- Our annual conference is a key opportunity for practitioners to learn from other experts, network and initiate and develop projects.
- Educational events are made available throughout the year, including presentations (face-to-face and online), interviews and meetings.

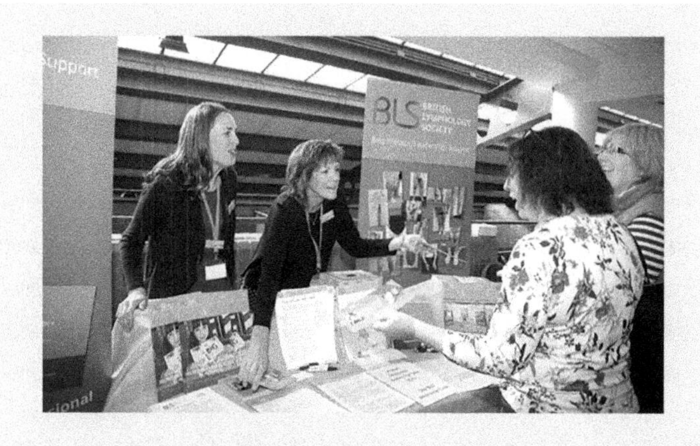

British Lymphology Society – Annual Conference

BLS is a mainly professional membership, for whom it provides a strong voice when required to advise or comment formally on relevant matters. However, anyone who supports our ambitions and make a real difference to people with lymphoedema, is welcome to add their support as a full member or Friend (at no cost). We are a small but growing organisation which is very active in producing and disseminating information materials to healthcare professionals and resources that they can pass on to their patients. We campaign with a particular focus on general healthcare professionals and the public during our annual Lymphoedema Awareness Week in March and have an all-year campaign to enable this information to reach as widely as possible, for example in our current EveryBodyCan Campaign (see Chapter 12 – Healthy Lifestyle).

To maximise the impact of our campaigning we collaborate with many stakeholders. By recruiting support for campaigns and collaborating with other professional and charitable organisations we are able to extend the reach of the Society and influence awareness and practice more widely. Current campaign partners include the Royal College of General Practitioners, Royal College of Nursing, Royal College of Podiatry, Chartered Society of Physiotherapy, Queen's Nursing Institute, Lymphoedema Support Network and many others. We are currently working with a number of charities to produce information materials specifically for their members and followers or to write articles for publication in relevant journals and newsletters.

BLS are one of the 8 founding coalition members of the Leg's Matter Campaign www.legsmatter.com which provides additional opportunities to highlight lymphoedema and other problems that may co-exist with lower limb lymphoedema. We also pool our expertise with partner organisations in other countries, such as the Australasian Lymphology Association.

Key stakeholders include all our members, whether they are healthcare professionals, people with lymphoedema, corporate partners or others. All are experts in their own way and we are constantly looking for ways to enhance our communication and understanding of the perspectives and experiences of each and how we can best work together to communicate our messages widely and strengthen the impact. As such I am delighted to have been invited to share some of work of the BLS in this book. For further information: www.thebls.com.

Top Tip #2: To find your nearest qualified lymphoedema therapist, visit *www.thebls.com/directory*.

LE&RN Worldwide Centers of Excellence

Centers. No, this isn't a typo. I've used the American spelling because LE&RN, Lymphatic Education & Research Network, based in the USA, has created a global network of Centers of Excellence. According to the LE&RN website "*The mission of the LE&RN Centers of Excellence program is to increase access to the best possible multi-disciplinary clinical care and services for individuals affected by Lymphatic Diseases and their families through a geographically diverse network of local and/or regional clinical centers.*"

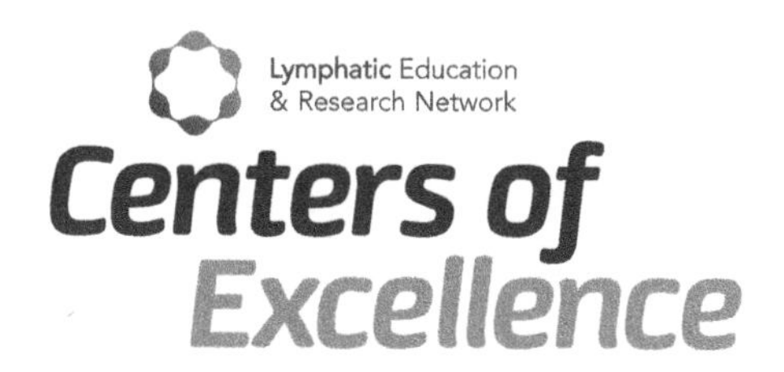

LE&RN first engaged a committee of expert clinicians in the United States to create a set of standards, which was then refined by a Global Oversight Committee to expand their global applicability. Letters of intent and full applications submitted by institutions seeking a Center of Excellence designation, are reviewed by the Global Oversight Committee. If these high standards are met, LE&RN award the clinic a Center of Excellence in the Diagnosis and Treatment of Lymphatic Diseases (LD). Professor Peter Mortimer is the Committee Chair representing the United Kingdom.

Of the 11 LE&RN LD Comprehensive Centers of Excellence worldwide, two are in the UK; St George's University Hospital, London and Derby Lymphoedema Service at the Royal Derby Hospital. For more information, visit the LE&RN website *www.lymphaticnetwork.org/centers-of-excellence*.

LE&RN President and CEO, William Repicci joins us later in the book to share his views of lymphedema (as it's spelt) in the United States of America.

6

MENTAL WELLBEING AND SUPPORT GROUPS

"Prior to joining an online support group, many people had never met or even spoken to someone else living with lymphoedema."

—Gaynor Leech,
Founder of L-W-O Community

As I mentioned earlier, for me the first year or so were the toughest in terms of dealing with this lifelong condition. Lymphoedema felt like such a huge burden that had literally changed the way I lived my life. I hit some very low points along the way, but, with the love and support of my family, close friends and Kelly Nickson, I was able to pull myself out of the hole. I've done a lot of soul searching for this chapter as I don't want to underplay the enormous effect that lymphoedema had, not just on my mental wellbeing, but also the effect that it had *(or I had)* on my wife, children and those closest to me. Equally, I don't want this chapter to be all doom and gloom resulting in you putting the book back on the shelf for another time. In fact, the objective of this book is to provide useful tips to hopefully help others, help *you*, to live better with lymphoedema.

In this chapter, I will introduce you to someone who has lymphoedema and took the decision to stand tall and make a positive difference to help others with the condition. There is a network of support out there, it's just a question of knowing where to look. I will signpost you to several places that may be able to help.

You are not alone.

I felt alone at the time, but in truth, I just didn't know where to look, or probably more accurately, just didn't *want* to look for help and I buried my head in the sand somewhat. It soon became very apparent, that I was not alone. You are not alone. We are not alone. Just in the UK there are an estimated 450,000 people living with lymphoedema according to Professor Christine Moffatt in Chapter 4. Who knew? When the time is right, it might be therapeutic to connect and talk with others who understand. It was for me.

One of the observations I have made over many years of attending several lymphoedema patient conferences, is the noticeable lack of men with the condition attending them. As an estimate, I would guess that the audience is made up of 80% female and 20% male guests, bearing in mind many of the men would be there to accompany their wife or partner to the conference and may not actually have lymphoedema. The first time I attended the LSN AGM and Patient Conference in London in 2015, I was one of four men with lymphoedema out of a total of around 100 people. That reinforces my point if nothing else does.

For many years I didn't want to draw attention to the fact that I had lymphoedema and was always too quick to respond with "I'm fine!" when anyone close to me asked how I was. I suppose I fell into the stereotypical "Men

Don't Talk!" category, which isn't sustainable without having a negative effect on one's frame of mind and mental health. No matter how hard I was trying not to, I was gradually becoming a grumpy old man. That wasn't helped by a complete stranger sitting poolside, whilst on a much-needed holiday in Menorca, asking me "What have you done to your leg?" and "Why do you need to wear that?". My brief and dismissive response was "I don't want to talk about it". Rudeness isn't or wasn't in my make up as I've been brought up to be polite and have good manners. I had taken the decision to uncharacteristically 'go for it' and wear my stocking with swimming shorts, disregarding my inhibitions and thinking "I'm on holiday. I don't know anyone here. Who cares anyway!" When this was met with only one gentleman out of a few hundred people, in two whole weeks, asking about my F'leg, I felt embarrassed and exposed. However, as the years passed, I got used to wearing the stocking while on holiday. If the same gentleman had asked me the same question today, my answer would have been totally different. I would have explained what lymphoedema was and been a lot more gracious about it. That comes with time and acceptance.

Ordinarily, I am a problem solver and will always try and remain upbeat and positive. Lymphoedema was testing me to the limits. At work it was suggested to me that talking to someone completely independent and unknown to me could be beneficial, so I gave it a try. I contacted a 'life coach' who *I* thought would focus predominantly on business related matters. How wrong was I? The life coach stressed the importance of me, my health and my state of mind, which can affect my quality of life and, in turn, the business. That was refreshing to hear.

After providing a summary of where I was, my first lesson was to focus on, and appreciate, the positives in my life, especially during the tougher, more challenging times. The exercise I was given, to be done at the beginning of each day, was to focus on Gratitude. I had to write down three things for which I was grateful and say them aloud, whilst looking in the mirror, repeating each one five times. This was way out of my comfort zone and unlike anything I had ever needed to do before, and I was very sceptical. How would this help? I'd look stupid! Who would see? Who would know? Worth giving it a try though, as it couldn't do any harm.

At the end of each day, the next exercise was to write a separate list of up to three positive things that had happened during that day. The following morning, I would rewrite my Gratitude List of three, some the same, some different from the day before. Clearly, the objective was to focus on the positive elements of my life that I was grateful for and pay less attention to the negative elements that were bringing me down. Some examples included the obvious, my wife, family, friends. However, I had to think outside of the box and open my eyes to what else was around me. It was pushing my boundaries to be sure, but it started to work for me. I began to appreciate many things that were right in front of me, but I hadn't taken the time to look.

- I went for a walk at lunchtime and actually stopped to look at the local architecture
- I would lay down for a while on the grass in the park and look up at the sky, sometimes just close my eyes for 10 minutes
- I'd notice trees, flowers, birds, wildlife
- I would have lunch sitting by the river, just watching the world go by
- I would play a round of golf at a relaxed pace, enjoying each hole and not getting frustrated if I duffed my shot. Who cares?
- I would relax my mind, forget about the stresses of work and lymphoedema and just take in my surroundings
- I slowed down my pace of life and appreciated the simpler things, like listening to chill-out or classical music
- I would read a book. I'm a big fan of James Patterson books, especially the Alex Cross novels

Previously, my excuse for not doing any of this was a lack of time, yet I was in charge of my diary. Instead of eating lunch at my desk, I decided to get out of the office and take a break, get some fresh air and jump off the wheel for a while. I have to say it actually worked for me. It focused my mind on the bigger picture again, which actually meant putting lymphoedema back into perspective. I was alive, I was fit and healthy, I had a loving wife and family, some great friends, a profitable business and I was able to take some time for me, whether that was 30 minutes, an hour, or several hours depending on the day. Things could be a lot worse, couldn't they?

Top Tip #3: Write a Gratitude List of 3 things that you are grateful for every day. Say them to yourself in the mirror every morning. Go on, give it a try, nothing to lose, right?

Top Tip #4: Get some fresh air, go for a walk and appreciate your natural surroundings. Nature is calming and therapeutic.

It was time for me to control the lymphoedema and not allow the lymphoedema to control me any longer.

As I said earlier, when the time is right for you, it really can help to connect and talk with others who understand. In 2015, the time was right for me.

Having lymphoedema isn't something one shouts about. Instead, I have done as much as I possibly can to hide my unsightly F'leg. It took four years before I was able to put my head above the parapet. When I did, I really wanted to make a difference and help others suffering from lymphoedema, including fundraising and increasing awareness of the disease. I wrote an article for the LSN Lymphline magazine Winter 2015 issue and then joined the LSN as a trustee soon after that, in 2016.

Also in 2015, I wrote a blog for the Levi's website about my experience with their Lot 1 made-to-measure jeans service. *http://www.levistrauss.com/unzipped-blog/2015/08/at-last-the-perfect-pants/*.

In 2016, I was a case study in the book "Let's Talk Lymphoedema" by Professor Peter Mortimer and Gemma Levine.

Early 2017, Professor Mortimer asked me if I would consider being interviewed by The Daily Mail – Good Health section and I gladly obliged. The purpose of the article was to highlight the number of men living with lymphoedema, a condition many think only women suffer from. This was published in May 2017 and still appears on the Daily Mail website. *http://www.dailymail.co.uk/health/article-4553390/The-men-left-agony-swollen-limb-condition.html*.

I was also interviewed by our local hospital radio station to explain more about lymphoedema. I've organised several events to raise money for the LSN and various other charities, totalling close to £20,000. I then decided to write this book and produce a patient-based website called *www.lymphoedemaunited.com* both of which aim to help people to live better with lymphoedema. I am also launching a Lymphoedema Support Group on Facebook, called LymphUnited, with the objective of uniting people living with lymphoedema and their partners, to share their experiences and concerns. I've reached the point in my life where I'm all in!

A few years ago, I was introduced to a wonderful lady who is also 'all in' since she got lymphoedema around the same time as me. She has created websites, support groups and a large following on social media, all with the main objective of raising awareness of lymphoedema and providing helpful information to those living with the condition. I am, of course, talking about the incredible Gaynor Leech, the founder of Lymph-What-Oedema (L-W-O). Gaynor has agreed to write about the importance of mental wellbeing, positive attitude and connecting with others in the lymphoedema community, through, amongst other things, online support groups and forums.

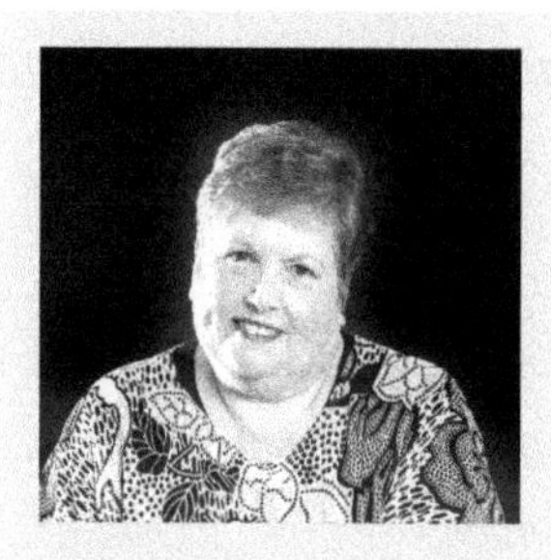

Gaynor Leech
Founder of L-W-O Community since 2013,
Patient Advocate, Self-Care Champion, Author, Blogger,
Patient Representative European Patient Advocacy Group

In the time I have been running L-W-O Community I have met many amazing people all of whom are passionate about the lymphoedema community. I was introduced to Matt Hazledine at the LSN Conference at Edgbaston in 2018 and have since spoken on the phone and exchanged several emails. I am delighted to contribute to his book and support the work he does to inform and educate those of us who live with lymphoedema.

L-W-O Community is an independent not for profit patient association, that offers non-medical advice and support accessible to any person who has Primary, Secondary Lymphoedema or Lymphatic Malformations their carers', family, or friends.

We have two online support groups and two websites that are aimed at both adults diagnosed with lymphoedema and families whose children are born with or develop lymphoedema in their teens. For anyone over 18 years of age you will find our Support Group at: https://www.facebook.com/groups/LWOSupportGroup this is a private support group. The website covers all aspects of lymphoedema, and the URL is https://lymph-what-oedema.com/

Our private Families Support Group you will find at: https://www.facebook.com/groups/lwocommunity4families In addition the website aimed at families whose children live with lymphoedema was published in 2020 and the URL is: https://lwocommunity4families.com/

Our social media presence is now 4,000 plus and includes members, followers, and supporters. They range from those living with lymphoedema or lymphatic malformations their carers', family, and friends in addition to those working within the lymphoedema community.

How did we evolve?

Late 2010 I was diagnosed with Breast Cancer through a routine Mammogram. My breast cancer was not a lump it was in the tissue it would not have been found without the mammogram at such an early stage. To all intents and purposes my long-term prognosis was good, I had a small operation to remove the offending tissue and 15 days of radiotherapy to mop up any remaining cells.

I was not told that the radiotherapy while killing off the cancer cells would cause another problem and I would end up being diagnosed with the lifelong and incurable condition of lymphoedema. At the time of my diagnosis there was little help, support, or information that would help me understand my new diagnosis. Disbelief and anger, I felt doomed. Through self-care I have learnt to manage my lymphoedema. My anger turned to a passion to improve not only my life but the lives of other people who were diagnosed with lymphoedema.

After being diagnosed with lymphoedema, spending time researching and learning about my condition, I had identified a need for more support. At that time in the UK, there were a couple of small lymphoedema online support groups. The question that arose time and time again "Was social media a suitable platform for a lymphoedema support group"?

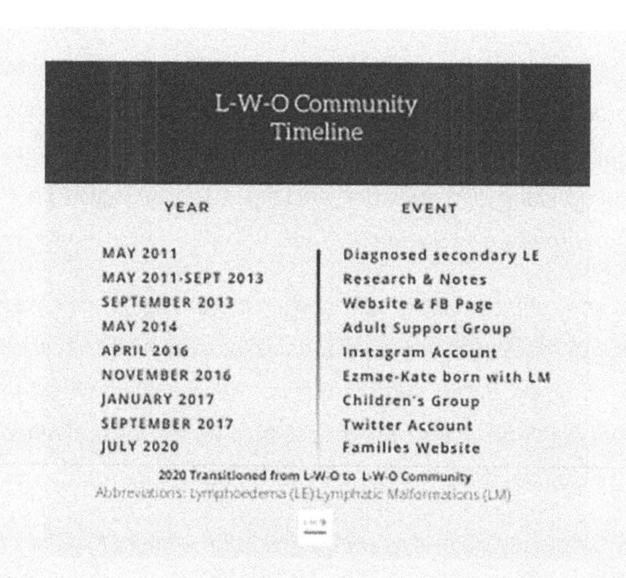

L-W-O Community
Timeline

YEAR	EVENT
MAY 2011	Diagnosed secondary LE
MAY 2011-SEPT 2013	Research & Notes
SEPTEMBER 2013	Website & FB Page
MAY 2014	Adult Support Group
APRIL 2016	Instagram Account
NOVEMBER 2016	Ezmae-Kate born with LM
JANUARY 2017	Children's Group
SEPTEMBER 2017	Twitter Account
JULY 2020	Families Website

2020 Transitioned from L-W-O to L-W-O Community
Abbreviations: Lymphoedema (LE) Lymphatic Malformations (LM)

Lymph-What-Oedema Community - Timeline

What are the advantages of belonging to an online support group?

Online support groups are run by patients for patients, that live with lymphoedema. Support groups like L-W-O Community have a global reach this means someone is available to chat online 24/7 365 days of the year. Sometimes it is as simple as having someone else to chat to who understands the daily challenges because they live with lymphoedema. Sharing their stories is not only cathartic for our members it empowers them.

We encourage our members not only to look after their physical health but their mental health. Our online platforms give support, we listen, allow a rant, and never judge. Prior to joining an online support group many people had never met or even spoken to someone else living with lymphoedema.

To join our support groups is a simple process, we ask two simple questions and once these questions are answered the request is accepted.

Myself as Admin, or one of our Moderators will welcome new members to the group our members will often say 'Hello' which then opens new conversations. Often members will open a conversation by saying "This might sound like a silly question" and our response would be "There is no such thing as a silly question".

We offer non-medical support often when there is no other help available. Many of us feel the system from diagnosis to treatment plans and support have let us down. Sadly, treatment is not always available on the NHS. We do not diagnose and wherever possible we signpost to other lymphoedema organisations when a query falls outside our remit.

L-W-O Community's aim is to encourage our members to make informed choices and encourage them to become their own advocates. We could produce fact sheets however with our main website and our family's website you will find the information all in one place. The L-W-O Community websites are written by me Gaynor Leech they are written entirely from a patient's point of view and they are not intended to be a substitute for independent medical advice. I am a patient, I learn as a patient, I read as a patient, I speak as a patient and I write as a patient.

Finally, through our online posters, presentations, and videos, we can educate, inform, raise awareness of lymphoedema most importantly we are there to support those living with this condition.

Thank you, Gaynor, that was very insightful indeed.

Top Tip #5: Connect with other people with lymphoedema by joining online support groups. Also, try to meet others in person at local support group meetings. Ask your therapist for information.

Of course, having lymphoedema affects us physically and emotionally. It can trigger many unwanted emotions including anger, self-pity, depression, sadness, anger, low self-esteem, lethargy, lack of confidence, anger, feelings of inferiority, sleep disturbance, anxiety, oh, and did I mention anger?

The LSN has produced an excellent fact sheet covering this in more detail called "Emotional and social aspects of lymphoedema". Fact sheets are free to LSN members. For more information visit *www.lymphodema.org*.

The NHS has also provided information and advice on *www.nhs.uk/mental-health/self-help* with 5 steps to mental wellbeing:

1. Connect with other people
2. Be physically active
3. Learn new skills
4. Give to others
5. Pay attention to the present moment (mindfulness)

The NHS has produced some wonderful advice for us all and it's definitely worth taking some time to visit *www.nhs.uk/live-well* and read the sections on:

- 5 steps to mental wellbeing
- Healthy weight
- Exercise
- Sleep and tiredness
- Eat well
- Alcohol support
- Quit smoking
- Healthy body
- Sexual health

Clearly there is a great deal of information freely available to us all, it's just a question of knowing where to look. I hope these examples have been useful to you and I know that we all have our part to play with improving our knowledge so that we can support our medical professionals with our self-care.

One area that hasn't yet been covered is sexual relationships. Sex is an important aspect of any meaningful relationship and can play a significant part in boosting self-confidence and improving one's wellbeing. I am fortunate in that I have a very understanding wife, who from the outset of me getting lymphoedema, has been nothing other than supportive. Her first piece of advice to me early on, was that it was perhaps a case of coming to terms with it and living with 'the new normal.' In the early months, my left leg was 56% bigger than the other one and it was a burden lugging this heavy weight around. My energy levels weren't as high as normal and I was lacking in self-esteem, which naturally affects libido and sexual confidence. Put it this way, I had never imagined that I would be the one wearing stockings in the bedroom!

However, where there is a will there is a way. It gave us the perfect excuse to experiment with different positions and have some fun with it. My wife said she could only see me and not my large, swollen leg. It wasn't long before my confidence returned and I was content with putting the light on again and taking her blindfold off!

I jest, of course. That's what we Brits do when talking about sex. We either make light of the subject or ignore it completely. What helped me and may well help others, was addressing this subject with my partner. You may find it helpful to discuss your concerns, what you feel your limitations are and what you feel comfortable with. If normal intercourse isn't possible due to discomfort or limitations, then you could seek alternative methods of enjoying each other. As you are in a relationship together, you should work on finding the right solutions together. After all, sex should be fun and not a chore.

In appendix IV there is a list of helplines and support groups should you require further assistance or information.

7

PATIENT SUPPORT

> *"The top priority for people living with lymphoedema is greater awareness and understanding of the condition among GPs and other healthcare professionals."*
>
> —The LSN

As explained in Chapter 6, it is important to connect with other people with lymphoedema and support groups definitely have a role to play. Patient-based websites like *www.LymphoedemaUnited.com* , *www.Lymph-What-Oedema.com* , *www.legsmatter.org* and *www.legclub.org* provide helpful information and tips for people living with lymphoedema. As they are usually free of charge to join, why not sign up with all of them to benefit from their knowledge?

Top Tip #6: Visit patient-based websites and sign up for newsletters and/or join as a free member: lymphoedemaunited.com, legsmatter.org, lymph-what-oedema.com and legclub.org

Of course, I cannot fail to mention the most well-known organisation that has been providing support and information for people with lymphoedema for over 30 years. I am referring to the incredible patient-run charity, the Lymphoedema Support Network or LSN, as they are known.

In 2014, during one of my six-monthly appointments with Professor Mortimer at St George's Hospital, we were talking about the fundraising that I was doing to support my local lymphoedema clinic based at Hospice in the Weald. Professor Mortimer suggested that I should also contact the LSN to see what I could do to support them, perhaps by writing a patient story in their Lymphline Newsletter. I had already joined the LSN as a member prior to his suggestion, but I hadn't been ready to put my head above the parapet and talk so openly about my lymphoedema, especially in a publication that was issued to thousands of people. Plus, who would be interested in *my* story?

In 2015 I was ready, willing and actually had something meaningful to share, in the hope it helped someone else with lymphoedema. The story I shared was about clothing solutions, in particular trousers and jeans. Normally, I would have to buy an enormous waist size so that they would fit my much larger leg. I looked like a circus clown. Now I had a solution to share with other leg sufferers. I go into more detail about clothes and shoes in Chapter 16 and provide several solutions to this problem that many of us face. I spoke with Karen Friett – Chief Executive of the LSN, asking her if they would be interested in my article for Lymphline. The response was a resounding yes, and Karen provided the appropriate reaction and encouragement for me to start typing.

The 2015 LSN AGM and Patient Conference was held in London, so I quickly signed up to attend, with two objectives. The first was to find out more about the LSN and the second to see the "Expert Panel" comprising Professor Mortimer, Professor Keeley and Denise Hardy, the LSN Nurse Advisor. Little did I realise at the time how pivotal attending this AGM would be for me personally. My first memory of walking into the welcome room was the amount of food laid out as the buffet lunch. Clearly, they were expecting a large attendance. The second memory was of one of the LSN Trustees immediately introducing herself to me with a warm welcome and asking me which practice was I from. I won't mention any names so as not to embarrass, but I was absolutely flattered, and when I responded that I was a patient, she replied with surprise *"Oh, I thought you were a GP"*. It appeared that the new clothes were hiding my lymphoedema very well indeed.

I was then introduced to Anita Wallace – Chair of the LSN and received another fabulous welcome. I really was taken aback, loved the attention and couldn't wait to hear more at the main event. As you would expect, the AGM, Q&A with the expert panel and exhibition of specialist product suppliers were exceptionally well organised and informative. This motivated me enormously to step up and see what else I could do to support the LSN. When my full-page article appeared in the Winter 2015 issue of Lymphline, it spurred me on further to stand tall and try to make a positive contribution to the lymphoedema sector.

Anita and the LSN team published a full-page article in the Spring 2016 issue of Lymphline, with the enticing heading *"Interested in becoming an LSN Trustee?"*. The timing couldn't have been more salient, as I had recently set this as a personal objective for when I retired, which at that time was 20 years hence. However, as the scientist and inventor Benjamin Franklin once said, *"don't put off until tomorrow what you can do today."* With that in mind, on 4th April 2016, I sent in my application to Anita Wallace and by 6th May 2016 I was working on my first assignment as a trustee in waiting. I was officially voted in as a trustee at the AGM and Patient Conference in Manchester in September 2016. I was absolutely buzzing and delighted to be involved with the LSN, in a position where I could help to make a positive difference.

Having successfully run my own business for many years at that point, I was able to apply my commercial expertise to my role as a trustee. I believe I made constructive contributions with new ideas to generate income and suggestions to make significant cost savings. One very simple example of this was folding the Lymphline newsletter in half, saving thousands of pounds every year in postage costs by using a smaller envelope. One of my many interesting and fun tasks was to liaise with the LSN sponsors to promote the 'Sock it to Lymphoedema' campaign in 2017, which was a great success.

The LSN Chair and Board of Trustees had recognised the importance of a strong online and social media presence to attract the younger generation of members. I was very happy to recommend the excellent web designer I had used for years in my companies, BeSmartMedia, to build and design their current website.

Capitalising on my fabulous relationship with Levi's Lot 1 made-to-measure team, I enquired as to whether there was any opportunity for them to promote or support the LSN. The outcome was that Levi's chose the LSN as their nominated charity for their annual 'Community Day' initiative in July 2016. This involves Levi's staff going out and helping with projects in the local community, in addition to selling discounted clothes to staff, with all proceeds going to their nominated charity. Levi's donated a whopping £2,806 to the LSN which would have certainly helped towards the cost of their new website.

I was always enthusiastic in this role and worked on several other projects with the wonderful LSN team. It is important to point out that all of us did this for absolutely no financial gain whatsoever, which made this work truly satisfying and rewarding.

Separate to my role as a trustee, I organised several fundraising events including co-running, with Chris Prier, the Firefly Charity Golf Day in 2017 raising an incredible £8,176 for the LSN. I also joined our local Christmas fair, where my raffle and tombola stall raised over £400 in four hours.

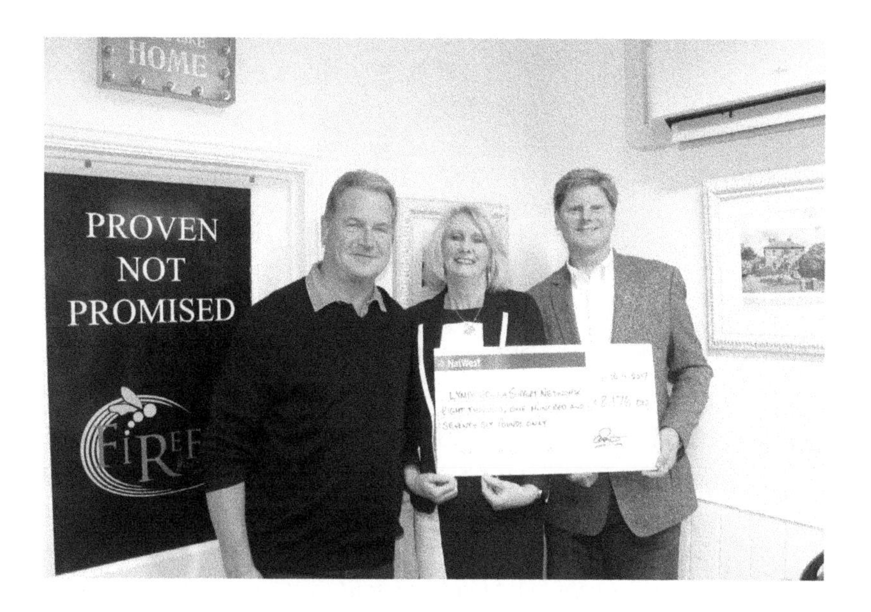

Firefly Charity Golf Day 2017 – Raising £8,176 for the LSN. Chris & Carol Prier with Matt Hazledine

After two and a half years with the LSN, I had to make the tough decision to step down from my position as a trustee. The overriding reason for this, was the time spent recovering from two intensive surgeries: Lymph Node Transfer and Liposuction, both of which I explain in detail later in the book. The recovery was having a huge impact on me personally, on my family life and on running my business. I could no longer commit the time I wanted to the role of LSN Trustee and it was with genuine sadness that I resigned my position officially at the AGM in 2018. This period of my life was incredible and really gave me the confidence to step up and make a difference. For that, I am truly grateful. I am still in touch with Anita and Karen, remain a loyal member and would always help to promote the LSN to anyone. So, if you are not a member of the LSN, add that to your action list because £15 per year is excellent value. Contact the LSN team today and please let them know that I provided the recommendation.

I am pleased to include a message from the LSN to provide more information about their service.

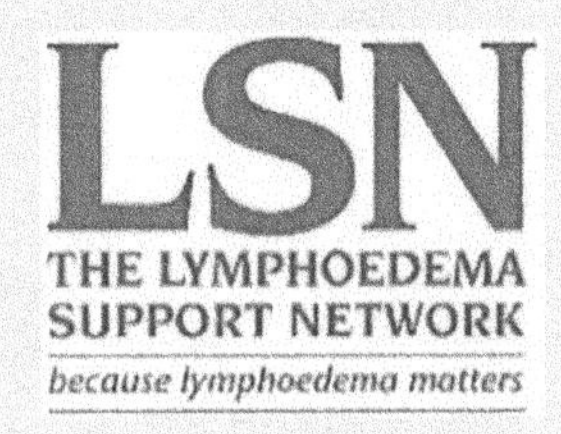

Each year the LSN, like all charities, holds an Annual General Meeting where the work carried out, our achievements and challenges are reported to our members and our aspirations for the coming year are outlined. Usually, the AGM is linked with either an invited guest speaker for the afternoon to make the AGM more interesting for those attending or a full day patient conference.

It was at one such event that Matt first introduced himself, it was notable firstly because attendees are usually predominantly female and secondly because Matt was very keen from the outset to see how he could help the LSN. Matt had a particular interest in raising awareness of lymphoedema, particularly among men who live with primary forms of the condition, he was ultimately invited to join the LSN Trustee Board, focussing on our corporate relationships and fundraising.

Matt brought another male voice to the board and it was extremely constructive to have this input and listen to his views, he was valued by all. Sadly, due to unexpected family and business commitments, Matt was unable to continue working as an LSN Trustee long-term. However, during his time with us he was able to share his story, provide some very helpful information and do much to raise the profile of our work with men with lymphoedema, he even found time to organise a very successful fundraising golf day for the LSN. We know that raising awareness among men remains Matt's passion and we wish him every success in his new ventures.

The Lymphoedema Support Network, LSN for short, has been providing information and support for people living with lymphoedema for 30 years.

Run by patients for patients, it has evolved into an influential and independent registered charity, providing a voice for lymphoedema patients.

It operates an information and support telephone helpline, maintains a regularly updated website, provides a Facebook page, Twitter account, YouTube channel and has facilitated a patient forum via HealthUnlocked where people can talk to each other.

The LSN is thought by many to be the largest patient information resource for lymphoedema in the UK and currently has over 20 fact sheets that carry the PIF Tic logo, the sign of an accredited and trustworthy information resource that people can rely on. The Charity regularly receives orders from NHS and private hospitals, hospices and lymphoedema clinics throughout the country. Also available are advocacy, school and care home packs. LSN holds the most comprehensive list of lymphoedema clinics in the UK, which is frequently updated. Contact information is also available for some private services and a list of MLDuk therapists is held.

In addition, a quarterly newsletter is produced containing articles on current information, treatment and research, as well as patient experience story's, hints and tips and much more. Bi-annual patient conferences with guest speakers are also held when possible.

As part of its work, to raise awareness of lymphoedema, the LSN works together with several other organisations and individuals with an interest in lymphoedema, regularly attends health related conferences to promote the impact of the condition and campaigns at local and national level for appropriate, equitable treatment for all.

The top priority for people living with lymphoedema is greater awareness and understanding of the condition among GPs and other healthcare professionals. In order to address this, the LSN funded and commissioned British Medical Journal Learning (BMJL), working together with LSN medical advisors to produce an online, multi-media training module entitled 'Assessment and Diagnosis of Lymphoedema' which went 'live' in December 2011. The aim of this project was to reach 2,000 UK doctors. The figures for the module continue to exceed all expectations; well over 10,000 individuals made up of doctors, nurses, pharmacists, midwives, educators and researchers from 123 countries have currently completed the module. Due to excellent feedback from BMJL, an increase in knowledge and understanding of lymphoedema has been demonstrated including changes in attitudes of the completers.

Following on from the undeniable success of this module, while the 1st module remains active, the LSN is funding the development of a 2nd module entitled, 'Management of Lymphoedema and Chronic Oedema in a Primary Care Setting' which is expected to go live in summer of 2021.

The fight goes on, join the LSN and add your voice.

Top Tip #7: Become a member of the LSN. It's a must for anyone with lymphoedema. Website: *www.lymphoedema.org* Email: *admin@lsn.org.uk* Telephone: *020 7351 4480* or *020 7351 0990*.

8

COMPRESSION GARMENTS, PRODUCTS & AIDS

"Many of these new developments will provide real and tangible improvement in the quality of life for patients."

—Tom Wright,
Director, Haddenham Healthcare Ltd

As you may recall from my introduction in Chapter 1: The Day My Life Changed, Forever, my lymphoedema was caused or triggered by a violent bout of cellulitis in my left leg in 2011. After 13 nights in hospital, I was discharged and told to go to the supplies room and ask for some compression stockings, with no proper instructions or rationale provided at the time. My wife, Vicki and I found the supplies room and collected two stockings, off the shelf, for someone of my height. When we asked for some more, we got a similar reaction from the person in supplies, as Oliver Twist received from the booming Mr Bumble. The response was a shrift, *"MORE? You'll have to ask your GP if you want MORE as this is all we can give you."*

I am now more familiar with compression garments than I was then, and I now know I was given a couple of Class 2 circular knit stockings with a closed toe. On wearing the garment for the first time, I remember feeling terribly embarrassed to show Vicki. I was wearing a stocking for goodness' sake! One thing was for certain, after the previously traumatic, painful and now life-changing two weeks I had just had, I wasn't prepared in any way shape or form to be told I had to wear a stocking. I loved wearing shorts at most times of the year. How on earth could I be seen in public wearing this? Mel Brooks' film *Robin Hood: Men in Tights* instantly came to mind. I wonder if I can get them in green....NOT!

I remember my first stocking with an absolute loathing. It barely reached the top of my thigh and it would regularly slide down my upper leg, meaning I'd have to go somewhere out of sight and hoist it up again. Very manly!

For many years I felt uncomfortable putting the stocking on in front of Vicki and would ask for privacy, while I did so. We are a fairly open family and don't like closed doors, but I did close the bedroom door while I struggled to accept my new routine of skin care and the difficult donning of my ugly garment.

Probably *the* most embarrassing moment for me, was after a large golf tournament. I had to undress in a changing room packed with men and try to hide while removing the stocking, hide my leg while showering and then hide, hopelessly, when struggling hurriedly to hoist a new stocking on with a semi-wet leg, without drawing any attention to myself. I cannot articulate how inferior and abnormal I felt. To this day, these memories are still very raw and painful to recite. In fact, I hadn't shared this story with Vicki until I wrote this chapter.

More upsetting than any of that, was the clear evidence that the stockings were not very effective as my leg was getting bigger with each passing day and week. My gauge to the increase in size was how tight my trousers were getting on my left leg. Pair after pair of smart trousers, suits and jeans were pushed to the back of the wardrobe, with most of them never seeing the light of day again. Many years later, I gave most of them to our local Hospice in the Weald charity shop, as they were a constant reminder to me of what I used to look like. Out of sight, out of mind. The same thing began to happen with my collection of shoes, which I could no longer fit my left foot in. Some of those I have kept, just in case...

In Chapter 16, I share several recommendations and solutions about clothes and shoes.

Witnessing the increased size of my leg, it was obvious that the stockings provided were completely inadequate in controlling the swelling caused by the lymphoedema. My mum, Annie, searched online to find a company that manufactured compression garments. The time she invested paid off and in a matter of weeks, the first one arrived in the post at great expense to the Bank of Mum and Dad. It covered my entire left leg and the fabric continued up to the waist and across into a pair of shorts, with a short leg on the right side. I now know the correct terminology is Tights One Legged Left. I used these for a few months but, unfortunately, they didn't control the swelling as I had hoped, although they were definitely more effective than the ones issued by the hospital.

As the size of my leg increased my self-esteem and confidence decreased. I felt powerless and desperate.

I bought absolutely anything and everything available to try and control or reduce the swelling in my leg, but what I really needed was expert advice on *the* most effective garments, products and aids to invest in. Kelly Nickson, Lymphoedema Specialist at Hospice in the Weald, was the person to help and in conjunction with the advice provided by Professor Mortimer and Dr Gordon at St George's Hospital, I would soon be kitted out with the specific products that would work for me. I was in luck.

Later in this chapter, I will provide an overview of the main products in the market that specialise in assisting people to live better with lymphoedema.

Firstly, let me introduce you to Tom Wright, Director at Haddenham Healthcare Ltd for whom I did some consultancy work during 2019-2020 to develop their new online patient shop, appropriately named LymphShop.com. Tom's main responsibilities include design, development & testing of medical devices and medical device regulation implementation. Haddenham Healthcare holds two medical device patents. He has kindly set some time aside from his busy schedule to provide some background on compression and, importantly, future developments in compression garments.

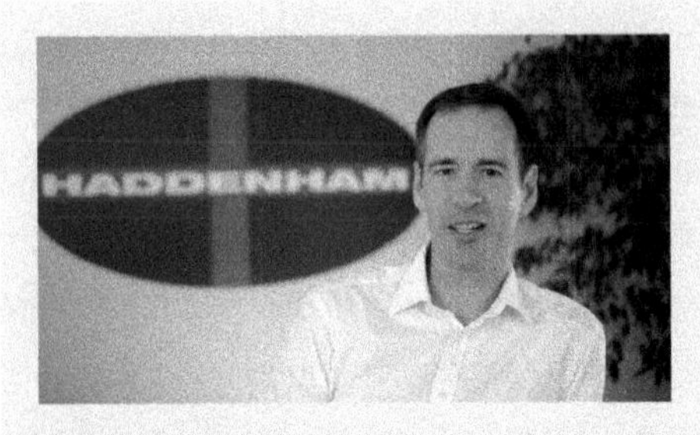

Tom Wright
Director, Haddenham Healthcare Ltd

I first met Matt when he was working for the Lymphoedema Support Network and was impressed with all of my interactions with him in that capacity. Subsequently, I had the opportunity to engage Matt as a consultant when Haddenham Healthcare were looking to build a patient focused retail platform for lymphoedema patients. Matt's diligent work ethic, business knowledge and passion for empowering lymphoedema patients was invaluable in helping to deliver a successful project.

Introduction and history

There has been a long history of using compression therapy in the treatment of lymphatic and venous conditions but until the industrialisation of latex, these garments were made with laced stockings and tight bandages with resin. Charles II's sergeant surgeon noted that using a laced stocking made of none other than dog skin had an effect on reducing a 'varicose ulcer'!

Indigenous peoples had been using latex for generations, it was not however until 1839 that this natural rubber had its first practical application in the industrial world. In 1846 the first patent for rubber threads was registered in England and this set off a revolution in the textile industry. A William Brown of Middlesex registered a patent for an elastic stocking with 'India rubber' in 1848; and in 1864 the Ganzoni Elastic Material Company was founded in Switzerland. A further development in elastic compression was the invention of elastane in 1958 by chemist Joseph Shivers at DuPont's Benger Laboratory in Virginia. This invention allowed thinner elastic yarns and today these yarns have largely replaced latex, although many compression garments continue to use latex.

Although knitting machines and yarn technology have come on significantly, current compression garments with elastic yarn all trace their heritage to this time.

Elastic compression products for lymphoedema range from bandages and 'hook & loop' wrapping systems, more commonly known as 'Velcro wraps' or just 'wraps', used in the initial phase of treatment; to compression garments such as stockings, tights, arm sleeves, gloves and so on, generally used in the maintenance and prevention phase of treatment.

Compression garments

There are three types of manufacturing compression garments. These are known as 'circular or round knitted' garments, 'flat knitted' and so called 'stitch-and-sew' garments.

Flat knit machines, and circular knit machine have their advantages for knitting garments with minimal to no cutting and sewing processes.

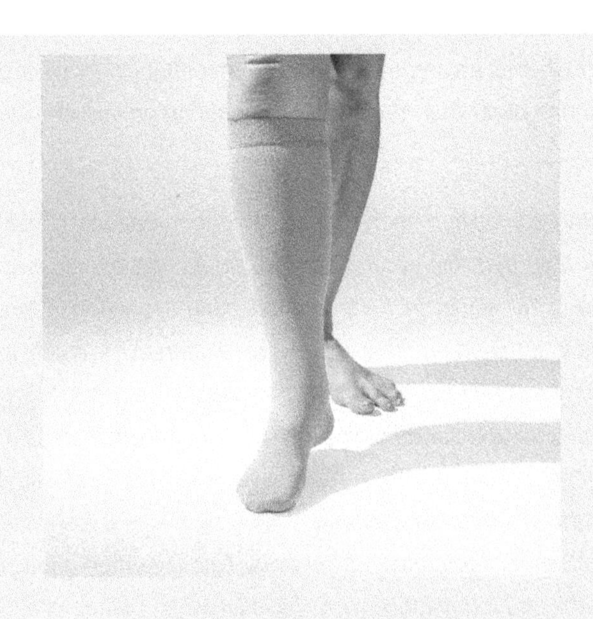

Below knee stocking with grip top

Circular knit garments are made in essentially the same way as a normal pair of socks. Circular knit products are knitted continuously on a cylinder to produce a seamless, thinner, more aesthetically pleasing garment. The technique uses less yarn than is used in flat knit construction and will typically have a higher level of elasticity. For more severe lymphoedema circular knitted garments may cut into limbs, resulting in pain and skin damage if used on limbs with shape distortion. This is especially true of some very fine silky stockings (like flight socks) which will probably not work best for the majority of lymphoedema patients and should be avoided unless used under close supervision.

Sometimes patients who are provided with a circular knit garment will complain of tightness at the knee or friction to the ankle fold. Due to the elasticity of the circular knit garments, if the item is not selected correctly or fitted appropriately, the garments can cause some discomfort. It should be remembered that circular knit garments can be suitable for the majority of patients who will not experience problems. Manufacturers are now able to increase the stretch in certain areas like the elbow fold, ankle fold et cetera in order to mitigate any potential issues.

Circular knitted garments are not able to handle very complicated limb shapes or hold severe oedema that may develop, for this you may need to look at flat knit garments.

Flat knit garments are typically less elastic than those made using a circular knitting technique as they are knitted flat on a machine, use more threads to provide a stiffer fabric finish. The edges are then sewn together to complete the garment with a seam along its length. Some lighter compression flat knits are able to be seamlessly finished. Due to their increased thickness, they sit on the skin better, resist cutting in and tend to be more comfortable. If your tissues are more pitting they can sit on the limb without constriction and are tolerated better by most patients. Although not as cosmetically pleasing, their performance and comfort are reported as better than their circular knit equivalents.

For 'stitch and sew garments' fabrics are knitted on rolls of material, then cut to the correct size and shape and, in a subsequent step, joined together, in exactly the same way of most everyday clothes. Most 'active wear' with low compression is produced with this method. For lymph-oedema patients these garments can also be very useful if a higher compression material is used; especially for treating the midline/torso region. One potential disadvantage of these garments may be the multiple seams which could cause irritation. In higher compression they can also be difficult to get on and off and typically incorporate zips, hooks and eyes, Velcro etc. Generally, the material used for 'active wear' products may cut in or may not provide sufficient support, so it is best to look for a medical grade fabric.

Hook and loop wrapping products

Despite its relative decline in recent years bandaging, especially when done by a highly trained professional in an in-patient environment, remains an excellent way to reduce lymphatic swelling.

Hook and loop wrapping devices have become more popular as first line treatment and management of lymphoedema as budget and time constraints for in-patient services grow.

Patients are also undertaking 'supervised self-management where they are taking control of their own treatment. The best 'wraps' for patients with lymphoedema would be those that mimic classic bandaging techniques which ensure a proper 50% overlap of the bands, graduated compression and allow you to wear them without interrupting your daily life.

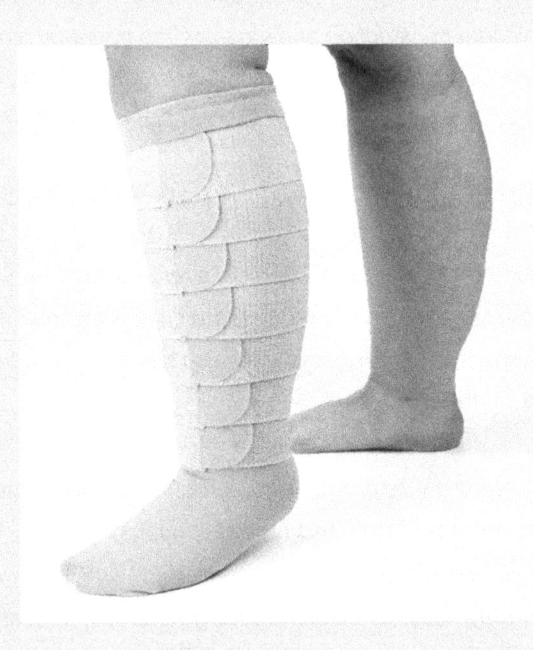

Lower leg - Compression Wrap 'Hook and Loop' System

The more you wear your wraps or compression garments the more you will get out of them, so those wraps which are thinner and can comfortably be worn under normal (or almost normal) clothing would be highly recommended!

Conclusion and the future

Manufacturers are continually developing more advanced materials and knitting techniques.

Garments are increasingly available with patterns or in colours which help them to look more like normal clothing. Knitting machines are also more and more able to produce garments with less seams and progressively advanced knitting techniques like 3D knitting; so-called 'smart textiles' are on the horizon.

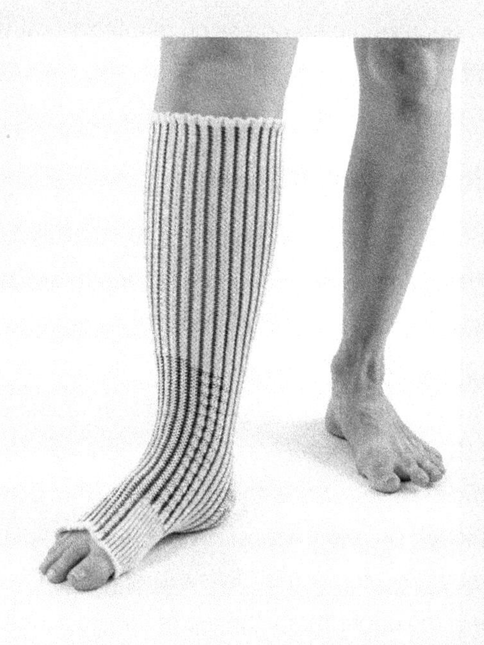

Below knee Comfiwave

Whether these new technologies will represent revolution or evolution is not yet known but from a personal point of view it feels like an exciting time to be working in the medical compression garment industry; and no doubt many of these new developments will provide real and tangible improvement in the quality of life for patients, which is ultimately the end goal of these products.

Thank you, Tom, for supporting this project. Like many things in life, one has to understand history to shape the future, and it would appear there are revolutionary technological advances in progress.

At my first appointment with Kelly Nickson in late November 2011, almost six months after being diagnosed with lymphoedema, my legs were measured. To my horror, my left leg was 56% larger than my right leg and the swelling was not under control by any means. She took immediate action to ensure that I had the appropriate compression garments that were correctly measured and fitted.

Compression Stocking & Sleeve

First on the priority list was a made-to-measure Class 4 compression stocking, with white silicone pimples around the top to grip my skin and prevent slipping. This was unbelievable to me, although perhaps not for many women who have worn hold-up stockings before. The type of stocking prescribed at the time, which I still wear today, is a Class 4S Jobst Elvarex Super CCL4 (60-90 mmHG) Thigh High (AG), Slant, Open Toe, Dot Silicone Inside – Outside Higher. I believe 4S is the highest level of compression from one garment, although on a few occasions I have been advised to wear a Class 2 on my lower leg, on top of the Class 4S, making a Class 6S. To assist with the drainage in my upper thigh, the top of the stocking is cut slanted downwards toward the groin area, rather than cut straight across. This works well in conjunction with the Eto shorts I wear, which I will come onto shortly.

I hadn't realised how many different styles and fits there were available for lower limb, including: below knee, thigh high, thigh high + waistband, tights for one leg or both legs and anklets. Additional options include: slant top, open toe, closed toe, partial lining, silk pocket, footless, no gusset, fly, open front, loose fit, Velcro straps, Velcro fastening and knee comfort (which I have in my stocking and it's so comfortable).

For upper limb, the varieties include: sleeve, glove, mitten (with or without thumb), sleeve & mitten (with or without thumb). Additional options: added shoulder cap & Velcro bra attachment, added shoulder cap & adjustable strap, a variety of sleeve grip top patterns, Velcro straps, linings, pockets, zips and slant top.

Basic colours include variations of skin tone, with most manufacturers also producing a range of statement colours and patterns. I have recently seen arm sleeves in the style of a tattoo sleeve, which is an extremely creative way of hiding the lymphoedema, oddly by drawing your attention to it. Is it a real tattoo or a tattoo sleeve? Dare one ask? What next - robot arms, skeleton legs, sleeves with images of bulging muscles? Remember where you heard about these ideas first!

Toe Caps and Hand Gloves

I have used a closed toe stocking previously, but my toes became swollen as there was no individual compression on this area. As I found out, fluid falls to the lowest point, so when my legs weren't elevated my feet and toes started to fill up. This was the main reason I couldn't wear most of my shoes at that point. To remedy this, I was prescribed Microfine Toe Caps, which are essentially gloves for your feet. The fabric is smooth and ultra-thin and each toe on the glove can be trimmed according to the length of each individual toe, providing effective compression. Wearing toe caps in conjunction with an open-toe stocking worked very well for me and quickly reduced the size of my foot, almost to the size it was pre-lymphoedema. Sadly though, not quite enough for me to reinstate my shoe collection.

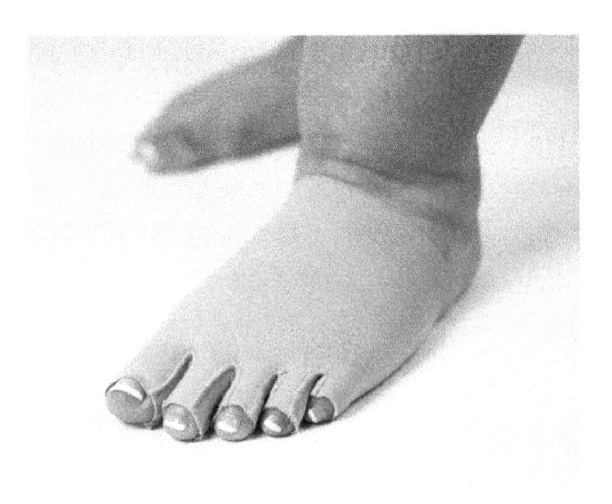

Microfine Toe Cap

Typically, I receive 3-4 toe caps every six months when I'm measured for new stockings. I wouldn't be without them, as they are an important part of my compression kit bag.

The same principle applies to the hand gloves. The fabric for each finger and thumb can be trimmed to size, providing compression for each digit. It can be worn in conjunction with a sleeve, if required.

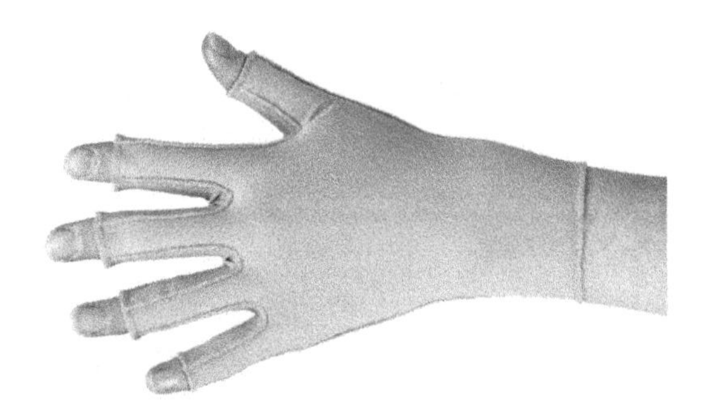

Microfine Hand Glove

Eto Garments

After wearing the made-to-measure stocking with the appropriate level of compression for about six months, I became aware of a bulge of fat/fluid that had gradually built up above the stocking top and around my hip area. I suppose it's comparable to squeezing an inflated balloon, the air has got to go somewhere, as has the lymph fluid and fatty tissue when wearing a stocking.

Although not instantly noticeable, it had become obvious that the fluid was struggling to drain above the stocking top, probably due to the issues with the inguinal nodal area in my groin. Therefore, the lymphoedema was building up in the left hip and waist and it soon became evident when compared to the right-hand side. We were just moving the problem and not entirely solving it.

I discussed the problem with my therapist and a potential solution was instantly presented to me. To assist drainage in this area I was advised to wear Eto shorts, which are like cycling shorts, but much tighter. I am very fortunate to receive several pairs every year, courtesy of the NHS. I wear black Eto shorts that are about the same length as jockey shorts. Eto produce a variety of shorts in different sizes, some that sit high above the waistline (pictured), which I may try in future.

There is a comprehensive range of Eto garments for both sexes. This includes compression garments for head and neck, bras, vests, abdominal aprons, genitals and scrotal supports, shorts, tights and full body garments.

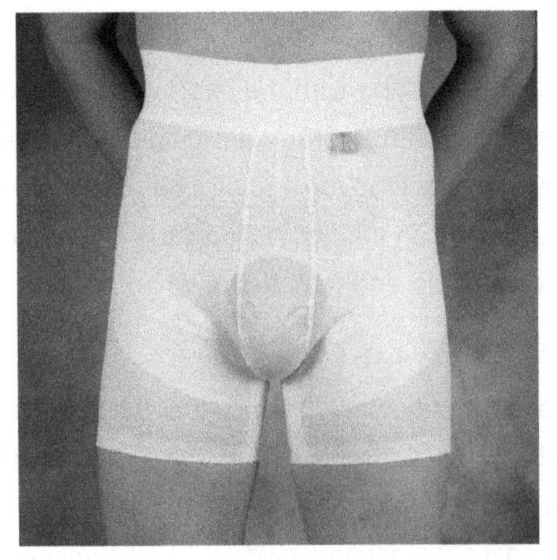

Eto 99 Shorts (worn by a model and not Matt!)

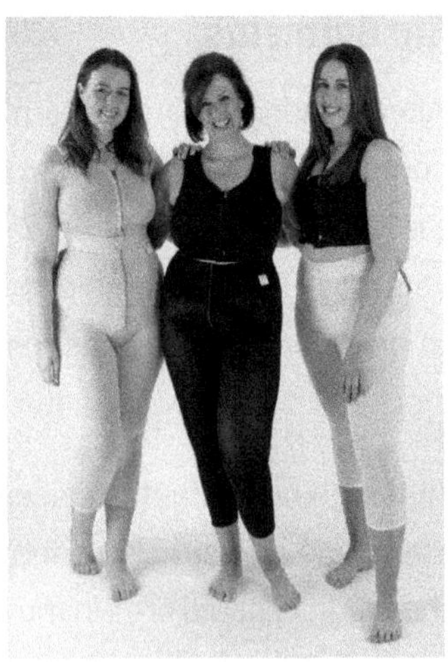

Eto Comfort Bra and Eto Grace Range

Kinesiology Tape

Another product that I was advised to try is Kinesiology Tape. The objective for me using this product was to assist the lymph drainage from my upper thigh and left side of my waist towards my armpit, where my 'working' lymph nodes should pick up the fluid and drain it in the usual pathways.

Clinics have used Kinesiology Tape for many years to help manage lymphoedema, particularly in areas of the body where compression is difficult to apply or wear. Taping assists with lymphatic drainage by allowing the fluid to move to an area that is less congested.

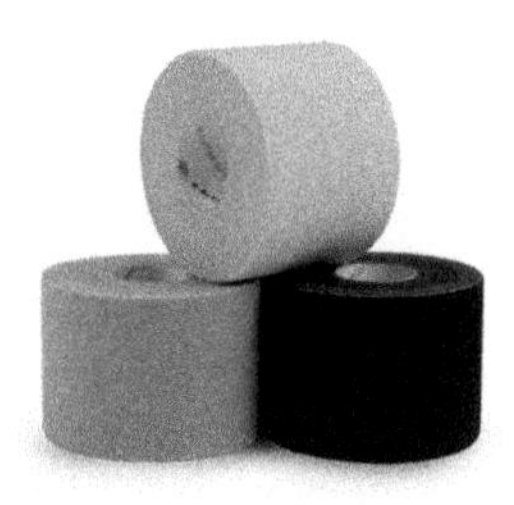

Kinesiology Tape

Mark Pearson, an MLD therapist first showed me how to apply the tape, so that I could continue doing this myself at home, as required. There are, of course, instructions and videos online. Just search 'Kinesiology Tape instructions' on YouTube or Google.

I first cut a length to size, from my upper thigh to just below the armpit, with a bit spare for good measure. At one end, I trim and round the corners, so they don't catch on clothes and become unstuck. At the other end, I cut lengthways along the lines provided for approx. 6 inches, so there are 5-6 strands.

Starting at the armpit, I attach the top of the tape (without strands), and peel off the backing paper whilst slowly attaching the tape to my skin without tension, smoothing it down my side, down over my waist and hip. Now the tricky bit. When I get to my upper thigh, I start unpeeling each strand and sticking it down, so it looks like a hand with fingers spread out. The ends of each strand should be below the stocking top, which is the start of the drainage channel. I buy a version for sensitive skin, as some brands I have used leave a red rash when the tape is removed, which can be irritable.

If you wish to purchase tape yourself, you can do so as a single roll or in a multi-pack. If you are in any doubt whether this product is suitable for you, please check with your therapist first.

You can read more about the use of Kinesiology Tape by specialist therapists in Chapter 14.

Donning & Doffing: Application Aids & Gloves

Now this is a subject that will be important to many of us who struggle putting on, or, to use the correct terminology, donning our compression garments.

I still remember the very first time I put on my Class 4 stocking, because these delicate office worker hands got an immediate wake-up call to the challenges that lay ahead. My knuckles were scraped and bleeding, my fingertips were tingling with the sensation of pulling on this tough, harsh, uncompromising material. I know, you have every right to laugh at me at this point, but I didn't know any better at the time. Getting it on was one thing, smoothing all the creases and rucks out was another. The material was like a cheese grater on these desk-jockey digits. This wasn't fun! Thankfully, common sense prevailed, and I grabbed some yellow Marigolds from under the sink in preparation for the next encounter with my Jobst Elvarex stocking. That was so much easier and my bare-knuckle boxer hands soon repaired to being fairy-soft again.

However, the rubber gloves soon wore out at the knuckles and split at the fingertips and they became an all too regular purchase on our shopping list. Searching online for rubber gloves resulted in many images that were quite eye-opening and not for further discussion in this book, that's for sure! Over the years I have bought many different pairs of gloves in search of the ultimate donning aid for compression stockings. Prices have ranged right up to £10.

To help you to avoid wasting time and money, I would like to fast-track you to the most durable rubber gloves that I have found so far, which I paid a whopping £1.50 for in B&M. This is a photo of the label and my gloves for your information.

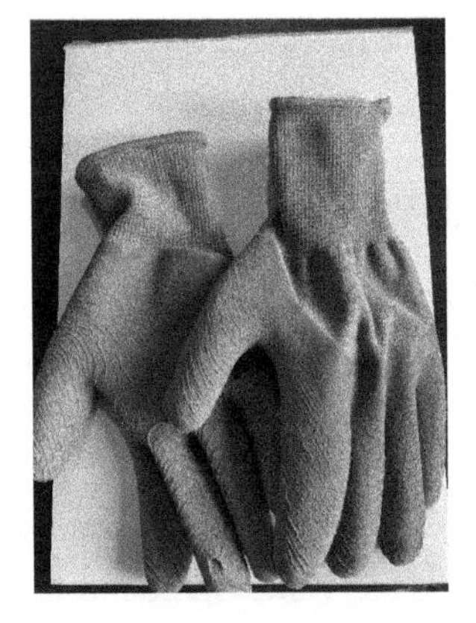

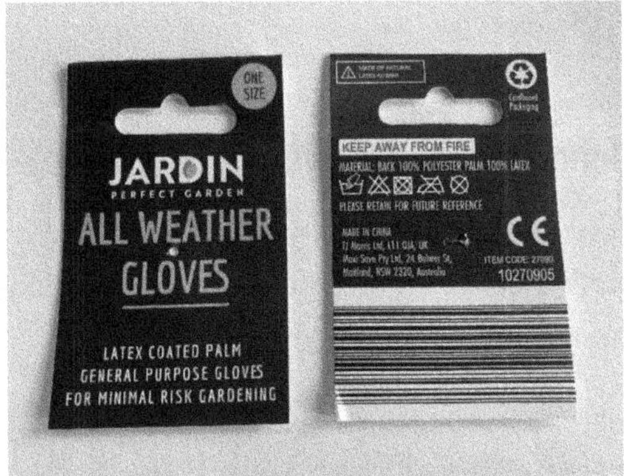

Matt's favourite gloves for donning - £1.50 from B&M

In case there isn't a store near you, I have found a very similar product online called Briers All Season Gardening Gloves for £1.99 from *www.charlies.co.uk* excluding postage costs.

I know that there are many variations of this glove available, and I have previously paid £7.50 plus postage for a very similar pair. So far though, these are my favourite and extremely good value for money.

Top Tip #8: Shop around for durable rubber gloves to assist donning. There is no need to pay over £2 per pair.

Of course, inside the bag of every pair of Jobst stockings I have ever received, is their donning sleeve/slider device (I believe this to be the case with other garment manufacturers too). I have tried this sleeve several times over the years, and again whilst writing this chapter, to see if I find this any easier. At this stage in my life, the answer to that is no. However, I certainly see the benefits of this method and clearly so do others, as various versions of this product are available to purchase from many of the specialist lymphoedema product suppliers.

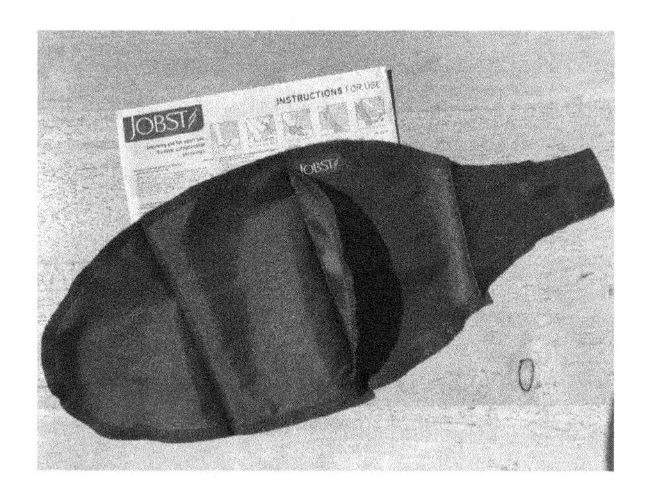

Jobst Donning Sleeve/Slider

For those people who are, perhaps, less mobile or agile there are donning and doffing frames and application aids that can be used whilst sitting down. Again, a variety of these products are available to purchase from the same suppliers. I understand from speaking with some therapists, that without these devices some patients would be unable to wear their compression garments at all, which, as we know, is counterproductive to successful management of lymphoedema.

Donning & Doffing Technique

I have watched a few online videos that provide visual examples of how to don a stocking, as I'm sure there are for sleeves too. One of the videos showed you how to don, just as if you were putting on a sock, which with a Class 4S stocking isn't that easy, unless you have tremendous strength.

Personally, I've never strayed from the method first taught to me back in November 2011. Perhaps naively, I thought this was the only way to do it but judging by the different techniques used in the videos, clearly not!

If you've got this down to a fine art that doesn't result in you breaking into a sweat, or breaking a nail, then you may want to skip this paragraph. If not, this may be helpful. Right, here goes my explanation. I start by turning the stocking inside out. I then put my hand inside the stocking to the end and pull the tip of the stocking back inside itself, to the length of the heel. I remove my hand, which would get in the way of the next part. I slide my toes into the entrance of the foot end and pull the stocking from the bottom back over my foot and ankle. The foot is now in the stocking and now I pull the rest of the stocking back on itself upwards to the knee, then thigh, using the rubber gloves to smooth out any creases or rucks and straighten the seam.

In my experience, it's much easier to take my Class 4S stocking off than it is to put it on. I have had a taste of how difficult donning and doffing can be when I experienced tremendous back pain. Due to the extra weight on my left leg my gait was out of line. The right (good) hip and leg overcompensated for the additional weight in my left (lymphoedema) leg, resulting in a disc bulge in my lower back. Reaching my toes to put the stocking on was nearly impossible, without lots of deep breaths and a few curses for good measure. I have often wondered how I will manage to don and doff a Class 4S stocking in later life, when I will not be as strong or agile as I am now. I took this as a taster for what older age may be like and I wasn't impressed.

Doffing is less problematic for me. I find rolling the top down as far as I can until there is enough material on the floor for me to stand on with my right foot as an anchor, while raising my left leg up and out of the stocking works well for me.

Again, this may be more of a challenge as I get older and perhaps that's when I will order a frame or application aid to assist me. Giving this subject a lot of thought, especially looking ahead has prompted me to start thinking of inventing an easier solution, which may seem like finding the holy grail, but if found, will probably pay off my mortgage!

Lymphoedema Products & Online Shops

As the NHS continues to finely balance their finance budgets, some of the products and aids produced to help people live better with lymphoedema may not be available on NHS prescription. However, many of the manufacturers and suppliers who provide these specialist products have created online shops to enable patients to purchase them directly. In fact, some also provide the facility to place repeat purchases of made-to-measure compression garments that have been prescribed on the NHS. As many of us are only entitled to two garments every six months, the washing machine is constantly busy and, after a period of time, the compression becomes less effective. With some companies, there is now an option to purchase additional garments, which are by no means cheap, but they are an important component of the self-management regime. Multiple pairs are also useful when on holiday and the laundry service isn't as convenient as at home.

These online shops are definitely worth a browse, as there are products available that will assist your daily life. Many of the products have been mentioned at some point in this book.

Here are some of the online shops that are available at the time of going to print:

www.lymphshop.com	by Haddenham Healthcare Ltd
www.sieden.co.uk	
www.mediuk.co.uk/shop	by medi UK Ltd
www.shop.lrselfcare.co.uk	by L&R Medical UK Ltd
www.healthandcare.co.uk	(type 'lymphoedema' into their search tool)
www.daylong.co.uk	by Credenhill Ltd

Top Tip #9: Research products available from specialist lymphoedema suppliers' websites and discuss them with your therapist or GP to find out whether they are suitable for you.

Lymphoedema United - Exclusive Membership Discount Codes

To complement this book, I have launched a new website called *www.lymphoedemaunited.com* which, as the name suggests, unites the core sectors of the lymphoedema community: the people with lymphoedema, the medical experts, the specialist product suppliers and the key charities and organisations.

Membership to this website is free of charge and, in addition to accessing the 'meet the experts' section, members will also receive access to a virtual shopping centre, enabling manufacturers and suppliers to showcase their products in one place. Members will receive certain benefits, including regular newsletters, and I am in talks with the suppliers to provide members with an exclusive discount code to redeem on all purchases made through their online shops.

This discount code will be redeemable on other products too, that will help you to live better with lymphoedema. So, please visit *www.lymphoedemaunited.com* now and register as a member free of charge. On registration, you will be contacted with a welcome message and details of the benefits only available to members.

9

THE IMPORTANCE OF PROPERLY FITTED COMPRESSION GARMENTS

> *"Regardless of chosen fabric, compression garments should never be "easy" to put on. It's a sign that they may not be effective for long!"*
>
> —Mark Pearson, MLD Therapist,
> Paediatric and Primary Lymphoedema Clinic Coordinator

Let me start by stating that, in the vast majority of occasions in the last 10-years of wearing compression stockings, they have fitted perfectly and have been surprisingly comfortable to wear. Although I have got used to wearing the Class 4S, it feels totally liberating when I take it off for a while when I shower or before I switch to the Class 2 at bedtime. As I mentioned in the last chapter, donning and doffing can be quite a challenge, especially as I'm not getting any younger, although I think it could actually qualify as a stretching exercise. I wonder if my therapist would agree with me.

The reason that I have received so many stockings that are correctly fitted and comfortable is down to the expertise of the two therapists that I have worked with over the years: Kelly Nickson and Mark Pearson. I say 'worked with' because I think that is an accurate description of a relationship between a therapist and a lymphoedema patient. We have our part to play in the self-management and in remaining compliant with the advice and assistance they provide.

However, I cannot imagine that I am alone in occasionally experiencing incorrectly fitted compression garments or even receiving completely the wrong ones, as mistakes obviously happen. I remember waiting for my new stockings to arrive, only to find that when I opened the wrapping, the stockings were for the wrong leg, which really does matter when you have a garment with a slanted top and a slanted open toe. Who could be responsible for the error though? Was it the therapist who completed the order form incorrectly? Was it the manufacturer for not following the therapist's instructions? Was it me for having lymphoedema in the wrong leg? Who knows, but the sad fact about this unfortunate and rare error, is the huge waste of money. I offered to return the stockings to the supplier but was told that they could not be reused and would be destroyed. I was told to put them in the bin.

It is very important to speak to your therapist if the garment doesn't fit properly, especially if it is too tight or too loose. I have certainly been guilty in the past of not speaking up for myself and reporting any issues. Remember, we wear these garments for six months before they are replaced and if they are not fitting correctly, it could be detrimental to managing the condition. If it's too tight it could cause pins and needles, or even numbness in your affected limb, and it could do further harm to your lymphatics. If too loose, then the compression garment may not be as effective in controlling or maintaining the swelling.

After my first liposuction surgery on my lower leg, which you will read about in Chapter 20, I was struggling to find the new compression garment comfortable.

It was rucking behind the knee causing the skin to become sore and inflamed. Naturally, I was concerned about the pain and that the skin may break thus becoming vulnerable to cellulitis. I reported this back to my therapist who was very happy to remeasure for a new pair. I wasn't treated like a fussy nuisance, instead he took the time to double check the measurements and discuss suggestions with me to improve comfort, including a new soft fabric knee band, which makes so much difference. I haven't suffered with rucking or pain behind the knee ever since.

Another issue that causes me extreme pain is when I get a corn on the side of my left foot, caused by the end of the open toe stocking cutting in and rubbing against my skin. On several occasions this has become so much of a problem, that even walking has been too painful. I didn't wish to bother my therapist about this initially, as I felt that I had already taken up many hours of his time after surgery, so I tried to sort this out myself. I used corn plasters, corn removal kits, corn pads, in fact every product on the market from all the well-known brands. I even went to a local chiropodist in 2018 to have them filed off over two sessions. What I should have done is let my therapist know as soon as it became a problem. But no, I waited until the next six-monthly appointment to discuss a solution for my next pair of stockings. Wrong decision! I remember being lectured, told off I suppose, and so I agreed that I would keep the communication flowing in future.

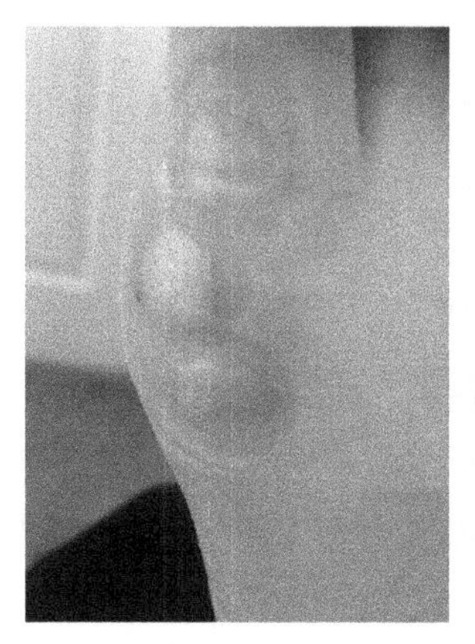
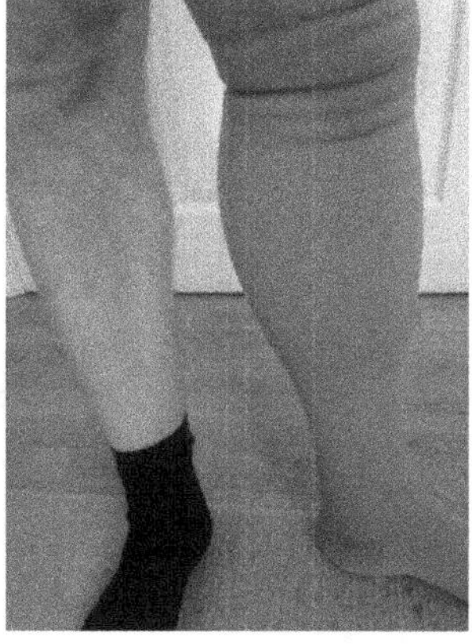

Corns on left side of Matt's left toe Matt's left leg showing rucking at the knee

The solution we came up with, was to give a little slack around the circumference at the toe end of the stocking, only by a couple of millimetres, otherwise it may have a negative effect on the compression. The outcome was that since wearing the new, slightly amended stockings, I haven't had a corn since.

Top Tip #10: If your compression garment is causing pain, numbness, discomfort, is too tight, too loose, not fitting correctly in any way, speak to your therapist as a priority.

During the Covid-19 Lockdown period in 2020/21, the usual face-to-face six-monthly appointments had to be replaced with remote telephone calls. My first one began with some questions about my health, any changes in my leg, skin, size, etc. As there wasn't any visible difference in size, we agreed to a repeat prescription of the previous stocking.

During this time, I did quite a bit of cycling, which noticeably changed my leg shape. My thigh seemed slimmer with more muscle definition than before, and my calf had got bigger. Sadly, this wasn't due to muscle definition, but more down to a lack of drainage at the knee. Therefore, I reported this back to the therapist at my second 'virtual' appointment. My usual therapist, Mark Pearson, was on annual leave so rather than reorder the same size stocking again which may be ineffective, I thought it would be proactive and helpful to measure my leg with my trusty Medi tape and provide more accurate measurements. The ones on file from my last face-to-face appointment, were pre-Covid-19, 12-months previous, which surely would be incorrect a year later.

I gave the new measurements and we agreed to proceed on that basis. When the new stockings arrived, I was keen to see if my input had paid off. After several hours of wearing it, the area around my ankle began to get pins and needles, feeling tight and tingly. I soon had to take it off and get back into the old one. I reported this back to my usual therapist Mark, when he was back from leave. Seemingly, I had measured my ankle at a different point to where the therapist would have done. It was completely my fault and I accepted full responsibility. I offered to pay for the new replacements, which Mark wouldn't hear of.

In my attempt to update the measurements for my new stockings and improve compression, I had caused myself pain, and, in turn, wasted NHS money on a pair of stockings that could not be reused. I suppose that is an important lesson which has helped to provide top tip number 12 at the end of this chapter.

Here's a couple of thought-provoking questions for you:

- What *do* you do with your old compression garments?
- What *could* you do with your old compression garments?

I pose these questions to you now and ask that you give some thought to your answers please, before we reach Chapter 23.

Over the years, I have taken my older compression stockings with me on holiday. If I am likely to go swimming in the sea or pool during the day, I wear the older stockings as the salt and chemicals in the water may harm the material and compromise the compression. I then change back into the newer stockings at the end of the day, ready for the night ahead. Does this justify a top tip? I think it does.

Top Tip #11: Take your old compression garments on holiday and wear them when you are swimming or sunbathing.

It is with enormous gratitude that I introduce you to Mark Pearson, my Specialist Lymphoedema Therapist based at St George's Hospital, London. As I said earlier, I visited Mark's private practice at the end of 2011 in a miserable state, with my leg an uncontrollable and uncomfortable size. He treated me with Manual Lymphatic Drainage (MLD) over several sessions, before applying Multi-Layer Lymphoedema Bandaging (MLLB) over a weekend.

Mark recognised that I needed expert help and advice to bring my lymph-oedema under control and reduce the volume. He suggested that I ask my GP for a referral to Professor Peter Mortimer at St George's and the rest, as you will read, is history.

Since then, Mark has been prominent in the treatment provided to me at St George's. He pays particular attention to how he can make improvements to the compression garments I wear, while ensuring that they remain effective and comfortable. Vicki and I are very fond of him and we have a great relationship with much banter, making the long trips to St George's even more enjoyable. Mark, a heartfelt thank you from us both.

Mark's areas of specialism are in paediatric lymphoedema, genital lymphoedema, MLLB and MLD. He will explain why it is important to wear properly fitted compression garments.

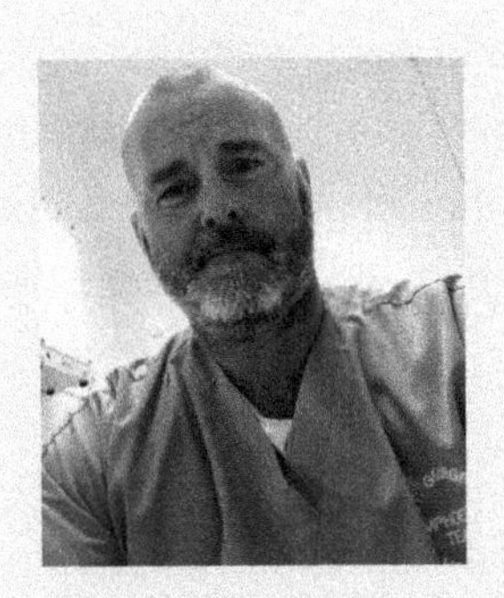

Mark Pearson
MLD Therapist,
Paediatric and Primary Lymphoedema Clinic Coordinator,
St George's Hospital

I first met Matt at my private clinic at home in late 2011, when he was looking for a MLD therapist in Kent. His leg was causing him great discomfort and he needed help to reduce and manage his lymphoedema. From my recollection, Matt had been diagnosed with lymphoedema at that stage, but not advised that he needed proper treatment (compression/

bandaging etc). Matt was desperately trying to find solutions and asked many questions that I couldn't answer, including surgical options. I did some bandaging (MLLB) but I knew he needed long-term care as Matt was serious about discussing all options, some of which were way above my level of expertise. I suggested Matt speak to his GP and get an urgent referral to Professor Peter Mortimer at St George's Hospital, as he is the leading lymphoedema expert in the UK. In early 2012, Matt became a patient of the team at St George's and the rest is history!

The importance of compression and properly fitted garments

There are several well-known cornerstones to effective management of lymphoedema. When you read around the subject or at every visit to your lymphoedema clinic you will likely be reminded of the following:

- *The importance of having a good skincare regime*
- *Controlling general weight and living a healthy lifestyle*
- *Appropriate exercise/mobility levels*
- *Manual Lymphatic Drainage (or self-lymphatic drainage)*

And there needs to be a multi-faceted approach but compression is key in long term, successful management of lymphoedema.

I hear objections already..."it makes me hot"...."It's so hard to get on!"...."I can't get it off without help!"...."It slides down my leg!"...."It rucks behind my knee"......"I get pins and needles in my thumb"... And after 20 years working with lymphoedema patients I could go on but you get the picture. And let me say – every statement there is valid and real and ***not just an excuse.***

Compression needs to tick so many boxes for it to work properly. Not just fitting well or looking good, you need to be able to get it on and off without calling for help (or breaking a nail!).

Good communication between you and the therapist who is going to be responsible for measuring you for the garment is paramount. It is essential that you really do understand your formulated plan. Your mind-set needs to be appreciative of the realistic outcomes from wearing compression – positive and negative aspects alike. Lean on the knowledge that your therapist possesses regarding compression and fill the gaps. You shouldn't be afraid to ask questions to secure true expectations of treatment.

Once you are confident with the plan and you know why you need compression you need to appreciate the science! These specially manufactured garments are made to ensure that when it is being worn your broken lymphatic system is supported and properly managed. This can be by encouraging the movement of fluid through the skin or re-routing it through deeper lymphatics. For arm and leg garments there should be graduated compression which means that the garment should not allow return of your lymphatic fluid to your hand or foot (tighter weave at the bottom of the garment when compared to the top). It can then encourage fluid to move towards the root of the limb and allow safe passage into your circulation. This is where the multi-faceted approach kicks in because when you start exercising or moving around with the garment on, you engage the muscles in your limbs and they work against the pressure that the compression garment provides to the skin. This is when the cornerstones work best as the lymph should start to decongest the swollen area. This is lymphoedema management!

Now it's all about you. You trust your therapist with their tape measure and you understand the way compression works. But why do you need it?

- *Are you expecting to reduce volumes (make the swollen part smaller)?*
- *Are you hoping to improve shape (correct shape distortion caused by the swelling)?*

- *Are you aiming to reverse thickened tissues (keep the skin from becoming hard and woody)?*
- *Is your goal to maintain volumes (prevent the swelling from getting worse)?*

The answers to these will determine the type of compression garment you need. (For example you are likely to need a robust fabric with a high compression class to re-shape an ankle whereas a lighter fabric with a low compression class may better suit for mild arm swelling.)

Regardless of chosen fabric, compression garments should never be "easy" to put on. I warn my patients to be wary of garments that go on too easily – it's a sign that they may not be effective for long! It is a matter of striking the balance between being able to get them on at all and appreciating a snug fit. If it doesn't lie like a second skin, it cannot work properly. There are donning and doffing devices available. For some patients these devices are the only way that they are able to get their compression garments on so if you need help getting compression on and off don't give up if the first device you try doesn't work. There are several on the market – talk to your therapist or look at garment manufacturer websites for ideas.

And we can stay with the importance of communication here because once it is on you need to be able to wear the compression comfortably for it to be effective. A garment that constantly rolls down, or slides, or cuts in or causes tingling or pain is not going to be tolerated for long. And you do not want to be marked as "non-compliant" so make sure that you ARE happy with the garment when it comes (length, size, compression class etc).

For some people, the aesthetic aspect is very important. And this is true for patients of any age including children. We all know that lovely beige/sand/almond/sesame/nude colour that Aunty Ivy used to wear but it doesn't necessarily mean you have to have the same. Most garments will come in a range of colours which may indeed make compliance less of an issue. Respectfully some people like to hide the fact they wear hosiery but there's a strong argument for styling it up sometimes.

In summary, whatever the compression class, colour or style of fabric you opt for, compression needs to work. Once in place it should not be painful. It should not cause skin irritation or slide and ruck. Getting it right can be tricky but it is worth the effort to ensure that your swelling is optimised long term. Work with your therapist to make sure that as many options are covered as needed to get the best garment. Listen to each other's suggestions and rationale so that the best solution can be put in place for your swelling.

Thank you, Mark. Through personal experience and reading your guidance in this chapter, I have to dedicate a Top Tip to this subject, due to its importance.

Top Tip #12: Only get your compression garments measured by a qualified and experienced lymphoedema therapist.

10

CELLULITIS AND LYMPHOEDEMA

"The LIMPRINT study already mentioned showed that those people, in whom the lymphoedema was not felt to be controlled, were more likely to develop cellulitis."

—Professor Vaughan Keeley PhD, FRCP
and Professor Christine J. Moffatt CBE

Excruciating Agony!

These two words describe my first, and most problematic experience, of cellulitis. To put this in perspective, I have a fairly high pain threshold and yet to this day, now aged 50, I have never felt anything as painful as cellulitis. The other surprise was how quickly this came on, without any warning signs. As written in the introduction, I went from feeling perfectly well, shopping for a new golf club, to feeling extremely poorly, curled up in a ball in A&E just a few hours later. I could not fathom how a bright red rash the size of a 5 pence piece on my shin spread so rapidly up and around my leg. It really is a shame that this photo is in black and white, as it doesn't do the severity and colour of the rash justice, but I hope you get some idea of the aggressive infection. I'll put a colour copy on my website instead.

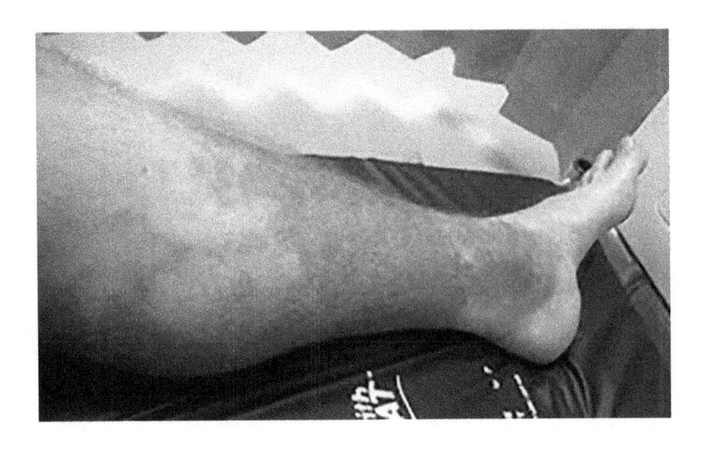

Matt's left leg with cellulitis infection in June 2011

I am eternally grateful to Vicki, for acting so quickly when she saw how poorly I was and arranging immediate childcare, before driving me to A&E at Maidstone Hospital that afternoon. Having read the NHS guidance (below), it could have been life-threatening if she hadn't taken me to hospital when she did.

Having had cellulitis twice, the second time in 2017, I am incredibly focused on looking after my skin and health, with the intent of avoiding any further episodes of infection. If you haven't had it, I genuinely hope that you never do. However, it's always wise to plan for the best and prepare for the worst, so I thought it useful to draw on the expertise of the NHS to share some very important information.

What to do and who to call if you get symptoms of cellulitis

I am quoting directly the following advice from the NHS website *www.nhs.uk/conditions/cellulitis/* so that if you experience the early signs of cellulitis, you act with urgency and get help, as the condition could be serious if it's not treated quickly.

The NHS advice is as follows:

See a GP if:

- your skin is red, hot and painful (it may also be swollen and blistered)
- you also have swollen, painful glands.

These are the symptoms of cellulitis, which usually affects hands, feet and legs, but can appear on any part of your body.

Get advice from 111 now if:

- your face or the area around your eye is affected
- your symptoms are rapidly getting worse – this could be a sign of something more serious like the rare condition necrotising fasciitis
- you have a weakened immune system – for example, because of chemotherapy or diabetes
- a young child or elderly person has possible cellulitis.

Early treatment with antibiotics can stop the infection becoming more serious.

Call 999 or go to A&E now if you have cellulitis with:

- a very high temperature, or you feel hot and shivery
- a fast heartbeat or fast breathing
- purple patches on the skin
- feeling dizzy or faint
- confusion or disorientation
- cold, clammy, pale skin
- unresponsiveness or loss of consciousness.

These are symptoms of sepsis, which can be very serious and potentially life threatening. If not treated quickly, the infection can spread to other parts of the body, such as the blood, muscles and bones.

Due to the seriousness of cellulitis and its significance for those of us with lymphoedema, I thought it justifiably important to invite two professors, both of whom are specialists in this subject, to impart their knowledge.

Professor Christine Moffatt and Professor Vaughan Keeley have collaborated on a report that caught my eye when researching online. Written for the British Journal of Dermatology, the report is called "*Cellulitis in chronic oedema of the lower leg: an international cross-sectional study*" which is available on *www.onlinelibrary.wiley.com*.

As you would have read by now, both professors have written in other chapters, so I am exceptionally grateful to both of them for taking the time to provide this vital information about cellulitis.

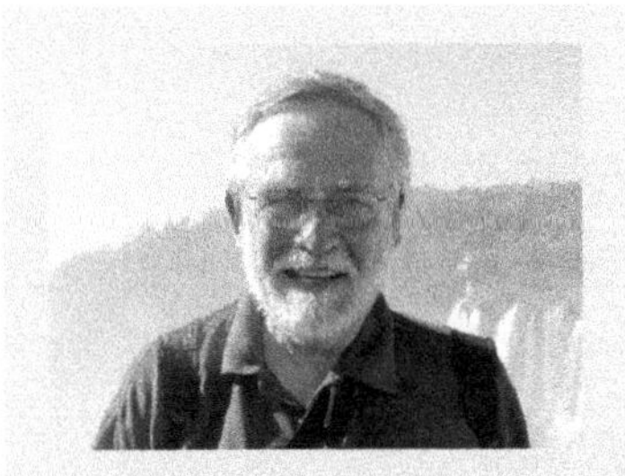

Prof. Vaughan Keeley PhD, FRCP
Consultant in Lymphoedema, Derby Lymphoedema Service and Hon. Professor, University of Nottingham Medical School

Introduction

I am a Medical Advisor to the LSN and met Matt at LSN conferences at which I have had the privilege to speak. I chair the LSN/BLS consensus group, which has drawn up guidelines on the management of cellulitis in lymphoedema.

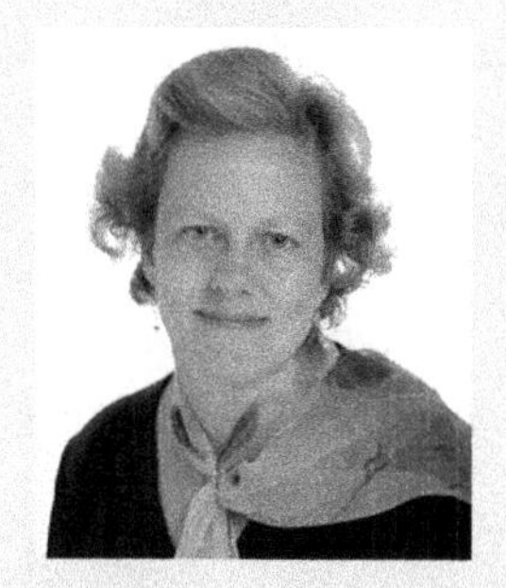

Professor Christine J. Moffatt CBE
Nottingham University Hospital and Emeritus Professor University of Nottingham

Introduction

Professor Moffatt is a nurse by background and has worked in the field of wound care and lymphoedema for three decades including with Peter Mortimer at St. George's Hospital for 20 years. She is a clinician and is particularly interested in showing how many people are affected with the condition and the impact is has on patients' lives.

What is cellulitis?

Cellulitis is a bacterial infection of the skin and tissues under the skin, which is a common complication of lymphoedema. In the recent International Lymphoedema Framework (ILF) LIMPRINT study, 36% of people who had lymphoedema of the leg had experienced at least one episode of cellulitis since they had had lymphoedema.

It can occur in all types of lymphoedema and in both adults and children. The LIMPRINT study has also shown that it is more common in those who have wounds, are obese, have diabetes, have midline lymphoedema (e.g. head and neck, breast or genital lymphoedema) and in men.

Some people with lymphoedema experience recurrent episodes of cellulitis, which can pose a significant problem and be a source of great anxiety.

The failure of lymph drainage, which causes lymphoedema also results in an impaired local immune response in the area affected by the lymphoedema. This results in the vulnerability to developing cellulitis.

In addition, cellulitis itself can result in damage to the lymphatic vessels. This can make the lymphoedema worse and in turn predisposes to further episodes of cellulitis.

Some people develop lymphoedema following an episode of cellulitis but it is now recognised that this may indicate a pre-existing problem with lymphatic drainage, which may predispose to cellulitis but may have not yet resulted in overt swelling. The damage to the lymphatics caused by the cellulitis may, therefore, tip the situation over into persistent lymphoedema.

What are the symptoms of cellulitis?

The acute episode of cellulitis is usually associated with feeling unwell with flu-like symptoms such as fever, shivering, generalised aching, headache and vomiting. This sometimes precedes the symptoms in the area affected by lymphoedema. In cellulitis, the affected area becomes more swollen, red and inflamed, warm to the touch and painful. In some people, the symptoms develop very quickly and the person can become very unwell with sepsis, requiring admission to hospital. However, for most, the infection is less severe, particularly if recognised and treated early, and can be managed with antibiotic treatment by mouth, taken at home.

How is cellulitis diagnosed?

In most cases, the diagnosis is made on the basis of the symptoms described above but, in severe cases, blood samples to try to identify the infecting bacteria may be taken in hospital.

It has also been recognised that cellulitis can be misdiagnosed. On one hand, healthcare professionals may not always be aware of the association between lymphoedema and cellulitis, resulting in under-diagnosis. Indeed, it was concerns about this that led the Lymphoedema Support Network to work with the British Lymphology Society in bringing together a group of doctors and lymphoedema therapists to draw up a set of consensus guidelines for the management of cellulitis in lymphoedema, the first version of which was created in 2005. In addition, it is helpful if people with lymphoedema who have symptoms of cellulitis remind the health care professionals whom they see that they have lymphoedema and are concerned that they may have cellulitis related to this.

On the other hand, some people with leg swelling experience episodes where the lower parts of the legs become more swollen, red and inflamed, often both legs at the same time and without any flulike symptoms. This commonly occurs in people with leg swelling, which may be, at least in part, caused by problems with high pressure in the veins. This can mimic cellulitis and is often treated with antibiotics, which are usually of disappointing benefit. These are inflammatory episodes due to increase in the pressure in the veins and are not due to bacterial infection, so do not require antibiotic treatment. They can be improved with elevation and the use of compression.

How is it treated?

Cellulitis is a bacterial infection, with Streptococcal bacteria probably being the most common cause in people with lymphoedema. Treatment primarily is, therefore, with antibiotics, given by mouth if the condition is not too severe but intravenously in more severe cases. The most commonly used antibiotics are penicillins - usually flucloxacillin or amoxicillin. Alternatives are required for those who are allergic to penicillin.

It is recommended that people continue to wear their compression garments during the episode of cellulitis. However, if wearing the garment is too painful then it can be removed but should be replaced as soon as it is comfortable to do so. There is no need to wait until all the signs of infection have settled. Paracetamol may be taken to reduce the pain.

How can the risk of developing cellulitis be reduced?

There are a number of ways by which the risk of developing cellulitis can be reduced:

1. *Simple measures to protect the skin in an area of lymphoedema from being damaged e.g. wearing gloves when gardening by those with lymphoedema of the arm and avoiding walking outside barefoot by those with lymphoedema of the legs.*
2. *If small wounds occur then washing and treating them with antiseptic solution is recommended.*
3. *The regular use of moisturisers (emollients) to maintain the health of the skin and its barrier function is essential.*
4. *Treating any wounds, skin conditions such as eczema, or fungal infections such as athlete's foot, which can cause skin damage and allow bacteria to enter the tissues.*
5. *In people who are obese, reducing weight should also reduce the risk.*
6. *Controlling the swelling due to the lymphoedema as well as possible with compression garments/wraps is also essential in reducing the risk. Although it has been known for some time that treating lymphoedema by various methods does reduce the risk of developing cellulitis, in the last year, two studies have reinforced this message.*

The LIMPRINT study already mentioned showed that those people, in whom the lymphoedema was not felt to be controlled, were more likely to develop cellulitis.

A randomised controlled trial in Australia found that using compression garments reduced the risk of developing recurrent cellulitis in those with lymphoedema of the leg, who had already experienced an episode of cellulitis.

How can the risk of developing recurrent cellulitis be reduced?

Recurrent episodes of cellulitis can be a particular problem for some people with lymphoedema.

In addition to the methods described in the previous section, the use of low-dose antibiotic prophylaxis may need to be considered. In the LSN/BLS guidelines, it is suggested to consider this if a person with lymphoedema experiences 2 or more episodes of cellulitis in one year.

There is good research evidence that low-dose phenoxymethylpenicillin taken by mouth twice daily is effective in reducing the risk of recurrent cellulitis. However, the evidence also suggests that the benefit reduces on discontinuing the antibiotics.

However, in clinical practice, if possible, the use of low dose phenoxymethylpenicillin is limited to 1 to 2 years during which time better control of the lymphoedema and the treatment of any skin problems should reduce the risk of recurrent infection, when the prophylactic antibiotic is discontinued.

If people with lymphoedema are allergic to penicillin then the situation is more complex. Penicillin seems to be a very safe antibiotic to use in low doses and at present the Streptococcal bacteria do not seem to have become resistant to it. However, the same is not true of many other alternative antibiotics, which may be considered for those who are allergic to penicillin. In addition to antibiotic resistance, a number of these antibiotics can be associated with a risk of developing Clostridium difficile infections resulting in diarrhoea, which can be very serious. Because of this, doctors are increasingly looking at ways of determining whether someone has a true allergy to penicillin or not.

As there is a general need to be cautious about the use of antibiotics to reduce the risk of bacteria developing antibiotic resistance, the decision to use low dose antibiotic prophylaxis is not taken lightly (so-called antibiotic stewardship). Ideally, low-dose prophylactic penicillin taken for a limited period as described here is the best option. However, there are small number of people in whom longer term, low-dose antibiotics may be necessary.

In addition, for those who have experienced recurrent episodes of cellulitis, having a course of antibiotic tablets to take at home as soon as the symptoms of cellulitis develop can be a valuable approach. If taken promptly, the infection may come under control quickly, reducing the severity of the cellulitis and avoiding the potential need for hospital admission.

Conclusions

Although cellulitis is undoubtedly a significant complication of lymphoedema, recent research evidence has confirmed ways, which may help to reduce the risk of developing it and, thereby, minimise its long-term effects.

May I take this opportunity to thank both Professor Keeley and Professor Moffatt for sharing their knowledge, in particular, how we can reduce the risk of getting cellulitis. If you haven't had it, I sincerely hope it stays that way, as it's horribly painful, debilitating and scary.

I recently had my six-monthly appointment with the St George's Hospital Lymphoedema Service, carried out virtually in March 2021.

In the follow up letter from St George's to my local GP, I noticed new additional generic content called **Lymphoedema Clinic: Management of Cellulitis Guidance.** This provides important information and advice to my GP, which will be held on my file, on what action to take should I get cellulitis.

I understand from Dr Gordon, that many lymphoedema clinics include this sort of advice in their letters now, which can only increase the GPs' awareness of cellulitis in lymphoedema patients.

Below I have used the exact wording taken from the letter. It might be worthwhile photocopying this extract of the book and asking your GP to add it to your file. I also keep a copy in my Medical Emergency Pack (explained later in this chapter), along with my antibiotics.

Important information for your GP, written by St George's Hospital, Department of Dermatology & Lymphoedema

Lymphoedema Clinic: Management of Cellulitis Guidance

Your patient is known to our department with lymphoedema. This condition increases their risk of developing cellulitis infections. The following guidance has been included to aid GPs with the management of cellulitis should it develop.

Prompt treatment of cellulitis is essential to prevent further damage to the lymphatics which can predispose to recurrent infections. Flu-like symptoms are often recognised by the patient before changes in the affected limb / area are evident. White cell counts and CRP levels may be normal, so please be guided by the systemic symptoms. Bed rest and elevation of the affected part is essential. Patients are advised to remove their compression garment whilst the limb is painful, but to reintroduce it as soon as it becomes comfortable.

It is believed that most cellulitis in lymphoedema is due to β-haemolytic streptococcal infection (Mortimer 2000, Cox 2009). The British Lymphology Society consensus group favours the use of Amoxicillin (effective against streptococci). Flucloxacillin is effective against staphylococcal but less effective than Amoxicillin against streptococci.

Always review response to first-line antibiotics after 48 hours.

Home Treatment

If possible, mark and date the edge of the erythema and record the level of systemic upset.

First-Line Antibiotics:

- *Amoxicillin 500mg TDS for 2 weeks*
- *If Penicillin allergic, Erythromycin 500mg QDS or Clarithromycin 500mg BD*

If there is any evidence of staphylococcal aureus infection, (folliculitis, crusted dermatitis or pus formation) then Flucloxacillin 500mg QDS should be prescribed in addition or as an alternative, if the patient is not penicillin allergic.

Antibiotics should be continued for at least 14 days or until all signs of acute inflammation have resolved.

Second-Line Antibiotics:

If there is no or a poor response to first-line antibiotics after 48 hours, second-line antibiotics should be commenced. Clindamycin 300mg QDS is recommended as the second-line antibiotic.

Hospital Admission:

Hospital admission for IV antibiotics should be considered if:

- *The patient's condition deteriorates at any time*
- *The cellulitis fails to resolve despite second-line antibiotics*
- *The patient has signs of septicaemia at the time of presentation*

Further detailed guidance including antibiotic prophylaxis, the indications for patients having an "in case" course of antibiotics and a detailed discussion of the relative merits of Amoxicillin and Flucloxacillin are available at www.thebls.com or www.lymphoedema.org/lsn/index

Top Tip #13: Photocopy the Management of Cellulitis Guidance section and ask your GP to add it to your file. Also put a copy in your Medical Emergency Pack just in case you experience symptoms of cellulitis in future.

Medical Emergency Pack

I was strongly advised by my therapist to produce a Medical Emergency Pack, as having had cellulitis once, there was a good chance I would get it again, which I did six years after the first bout.

These are the items that I keep in my Emergency Pack, which may not be right for you, of course.

- Antibiotics
- Paracetamol
- Disposable Thermometers x 3
- Pocket sized tissues
- Flexitol Heel Balm (in case of cracked skin)
- Antiseptic Wipes
- Antibacterial Hand Gel
- Cushioned Plasters (in case of a cut or blister)
- Corn Plasters & Foam Cushions
- Lipsyl
- Scissors

Please contact your GP and Lymphoedema Therapist for their advice on what is the most appropriate medication and items to suit your personal circumstances. The list above is specific to my condition only and may not be suitable for others.

Top Tip #14: Produce a Medical Emergency Pack, just in case you get cellulitis symptoms in future.

11

SKIN CARE

"Keeping your skin intact is the first line of defence against developing infection in the affected area"

—Kelly Nickson,
Lymphoedema Clinical Nurse Specialist

When I first met the team of therapists at Hospice in the Weald, they explained the four cornerstones of self-managing lymphoedema: Skin Care, Compression, Healthy Lifestyle/Movement and Lymphatic Drainage. All of these topics are covered in more detail in separate chapters. This chapter focuses on the importance of good Skin Care. A break in the skin can allow bacteria to enter, possibly resulting in a very painful and damaging infection called cellulitis, which I know only too well, and can result in hospitalisation.

As covered in Chapter 10, in a perfect storm of events, I had a pretty violent bout of cellulitis back in 2011 which damaged the lymphatics in my left leg causing lymphoedema. The perfect storm included removal of lymph nodes in my groin during surgery for a suspected strangulated hernia; a fall down some metal cornered stairs carrying a heavy oak table causing some significant bruising; and an open blister on my left toe creating a break in the skin. In other words, some of the key elements of secondary lymphoedema: injury, infection, surgery and trauma.

Prior to my initial visit to the therapist, I hadn't made any changes to my normal daily life and was still using my usual shower gel, having hot baths, using the steam room, sauna, jacuzzi at the gym, walking outside in the garden in bare feet and using a razor to shave my legs. OK, maybe not the last one, I promise! Fortunately, my occupation doesn't put me at risk of any open wounds other than perhaps a paper cut. It is worth considering any risks that your occupation may pose. It is prudent to discuss a plan with your boss or Occupational Health Team to put steps in place to reduce, or even eliminate, any risks. I am not at risk of breaking my skin in any high-risk, thrill-seeking hobbies or sports. The closest I might come to any harm is getting a blister on my toe from a new pair of golf shoes...Oh, wait a minute...!

Top Tip #15: Evaluate any sports or hobbies you enjoy, that could put you at risk of damaging or breaking your skin.

Top Tip #16: Perform a risk assessment at your workplace and put steps in place to reduce the risk of damaging or breaking your skin and getting an infection.

I have always listened to the advice my therapists have provided and more importantly, acted upon it. From personal experience, it pays to be as compliant as possible. The therapist is doing as much as they possibly can to help me. The very least I can do is to help them to help me, by doing as I am asked. I can imagine it is quite demotivating and challenging for a therapist to meet their patient at the next review appointment, only to find that the patient has ignored their advice and, as a result, is in a worse state than at their last appointment. The only loser with non-compliance is me.

Don't get me wrong, there are aspects of the self-management guidelines that either don't work for me, or which I have adapted over time to suit my situation. It has taken me many years to understand where I need to focus to maintain the current good health and size of my leg. Subsequently, I am in a much better place and able to better control my lymphoedema, rather than have it control me.

I can say with confidence though, that there isn't much I haven't tried to reduce the swelling in my leg. The starting point is always to try and keep your skin in good condition. Good skin care is so important to try and prevent infection, especially when you have lymphoedema. No matter what books, leaflets, websites, Frequently Asked Questions you read, skin care is consistently mentioned with utmost importance.

From the outset, my first therapist recommended Dermol 200 Shower Emollient and Dermol 500 Lotion for me to use daily. I order both products on prescription from my local GP. To reduce my prescription costs, I pay £10.81 per month via Direct Debit over 10 months (annual cost of £108.10) for an NHS Prescription Prepayment Certificate. This entitles me to unlimited prescriptions during the year. With the cost of a prescription currently at £9.35 for each item (at the time of writing May 2021) that seems excellent value to me. I would normally have at least two prescriptions per month, one for the Dermol 500 and one for the Dermol 200. I make that a minimum saving of £116 pa, without taking into account anything else I should need on prescription. Dermol isn't cheap to buy privately either. Online UK prices are between £8.49 and £9.99 for Dermol 500 and £4.74 to £4.99 for Dermol 200, excluding any delivery costs, of course.

Top Tip #17: Sign up for an annual NHS Prescription Prepayment Certificate and save money (if usual prescription costs apply and you are based in the UK, of course). *https://www.nhsbsa.nhs.uk/help-nhs-prescription-costs/prescription-prepayment-certificates-ppcs*

There are other products on the market including: Aqueous Cream, E45 wash and lotion, Neutrogena, Vaseline Derma Care and Diprobase to name a handful of examples. It is always worth checking with your therapist which product(s) they feel are best suited to you, before also checking with your GP and asking whether you can get them on prescription.

Personally, I am very satisfied with Dermol and was reassured to see that the same products are used by the team of lymphoedema therapists at St George's Hospital. Made by Dermal Laboratories in Hitchin, Hertfordshire, England, Dermol is an antimicrobial emollient and moisturiser for the management of dry and pruritic (itchy) skin conditions, especially eczema and dermatitis.

There are two types of 'active ingredient' in these products: benzalkonium chloride and chlorhexidine dihydrochloride which are antimicrobials. These help to combat bacteria present on your skin that can make eczema worse and prevent infection caused by scratching itchy skin, both of which are important factors for me, living with lymphoedema and trying to prevent cellulitis. The products also contain liquid paraffin and isopropyl myristate, both are emollients which help to soften, moisturise and protect your skin by trapping moisture and restoring the normal protective function of the skin. In addition, emollients prevent the skin-drying and irritant effects that can be caused by washing and bathing and by the soaps, foaming additives and fragrances used in ordinary skin cleansing products.

Dermol 200 is used as an emollient soap substitute in the shower as a replacement to normal shower gel or soap.

From a practical point of view, during my daily shower I wet my body (obviously) and apply the Dermol shower emollient all over my affected left leg and foot and then step away from the water flow, while applying my usual 'normal' shower gel over the rest of my body, trying not to get any on my left leg. After washing and rinsing my hair, I then rinse off the Dermol from my leg, having given it as long as possible to soak into the skin. The written instructions say one should "pat the skin dry with a soft towel (avoid rubbing as this can make dry skin conditions worse)".

After drying off, I then use Dermol 500 Lotion, which is an antimicrobial emollient and moisturiser for the management of dry and pruritic (itchy) skin conditions, especially eczema and dermatitis. I apply the Dermol 500 to the whole of my affected leg and foot, especially between the toes and then let the lotion soak into my skin. OK, I will admit that I can be a little impatient and often hastily put on my toe cap and stocking before all traces of the lotion have disappeared. Apparently, if this is done too often, it can have a detrimental effect on the material used in making the compression garment. As my garments are washed daily, I am not always as compliant as I perhaps should be on this point and should be more patient. Must try harder to comply Hazledine!

Using Dermol provides me with some reassurance that I am looking after my skin and creating a barrier to prevent infection, especially from the dreaded cellulitis. I do recognise that skin care is a very important part of my daily routine and self-management and it is now second nature. It is advisable to ensure that you place your repeat prescription well before you are due to run out of lotion, which during the Covid-19 pandemic and several lockdowns, has been trickier to arrange.

Top Tip #18: Don't ever run out of skin care products! When down to the last three shower emollients, tear off the lid of the box as a reminder to order a repeat prescription.

It is important to check the ingredients in case of a possible reaction or side-effects. They also contain liquid paraffin and cetostearyl alcohol and as a result of these ingredients, the packaging does feature a safety warning about the product being flammable and to avoid smoking or having naked flames near your skin. As you would expect, there is a lengthy information leaflet in the box, which should be read before using the product.

As I said earlier, my therapist drilled into me the importance of good skin care and I am pleased to re-introduce you to Kelly Nickson, Lymphoedema Clinical Nurse Specialist. She will explain more about why skin care is a cornerstone of self-management and provide guidance to help us to help ourselves.

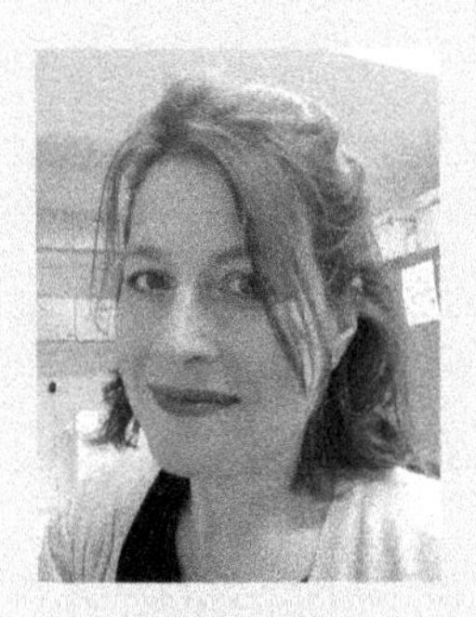

Kelly Nickson
Lymphoedema Clinical Nurse Specialist

Skin care is an essential part of daily self-management for people who have lymphoedema or who are at risk of developing lymphoedema. Keeping your skin intact is the first line of defence against developing infection in the affected area and looking after your skin helps it to perform this important function.

Lymphoedema can cause the skin to thicken and become dry, which means the skin surface can be more likely to become an entry point for bacteria which can lead to infection. Regular cleansing and moisturising to keep the skin supple and intact will keep the skin hydrated and in good condition, reducing the risk of developing infection which may worsen your lymphoedema.

There is widely published guidance on how to maintain good skin care, and you may have been given specific advice by your Lymphoedema Specialist or other health care professionals. Detailed information is available from the Lymphoedema Support Network and many cancer charities and is easily accessible online. Information provided includes:

- ***Keeping your skin clean***

  It is important to wash your skin daily but also to ensure meticulous drying. Plain water, or a non-perfumed/ bland soap or soap substitute can be used. Extra care should be taken to dry thoroughly between fingers and toes and in skin folds and you should observe for any signs of fungal infections in these areas such as itching, red, or broken skin which will require prompt treatment with anti-fungal creams or sprays which can be purchased at a pharmacy or prescribed by your doctor. When treating fungal infections on the feet, shoes should also be treated with an antifungal spray to prevent re-infecting yourself when you wear them.

- ***Keeping your skin supple and intact***

  Moisturise your skin each day by applying a non-perfumed moisturising cream or ointment. Your Lymphoedema Specialist will be able to advise if you require a specific cream, but most creams can be easily purchased via a pharmacy or supermarket or may be prescribed by your GP. When applying cream, go downwards in the direction of hair growth for the last stroke to reduce the risk of irritation at the base of the hairs. If you find it hard to reach to apply creams, then spray creams such as Emollin can be prescribed. Alternatively, long handled applicators or sponges can be helpful or even small, long handled rollers used to paint behind radiators as the heads can be regularly replaced.

Some perfumes and perfumed creams can cause irritation which can lead to increased swelling or breaks in the skin, so it is best to avoid anything highly perfumed and to patch test new creams before using. Avoid getting sunburnt which can dry the skin and cause irritation. Use a high factor (50SPF) sun cream or lotion.

- ***Taking care of hands and feet***

  If you have upper limb lymphoedema, wear protective gloves when washing up or gardening or performing activities which may lead to scratches or cuts. (If you wear compression garments, wear gloves over these rather than remove the garments.)

  If you have lower limb lymphoedema, it is important to wear well-fitting supportive footwear which covers the whole of the foot and prevents swelling accumulating on the top of your foot or between straps. Avoid wearing ill- fitting shoes which may rub and cause blisters. Use clippers or a nail file to maintain your nails rather than scissors to reduce the risk of cuts and if you are unable to reach or find this difficult to manage yourself, you may wish to visit a podiatrist for this. Avoid going barefoot, particularly outside, to minimise the risk of infection.

- ***Avoiding cuts and bites and breaks to the skin***

  It can be difficult to avoid insect bites, but some suggested precautions include wearing long sleeves or trousers to protect areas of swelling particularly if undertaking activities such as gardening or walking or hiking or foreign travel where you may be more likely to be stung or bitten. Use a good insect repellent making sure to patch test it first. If there is a reaction to the insect bite, you could consider antihistamine creams or tablets and your pharmacist will be able to advise regarding this.

If shaving the affected area, it is best to use a battery-operated shaver rather than a wet razor or epilator to avoid creating breaks to the skin. You can use hair removal creams, but these can sometimes cause a reaction, so if you use them, it is important to patch test them first.

Avoiding breaks to the skin where possible should also be considered when undergoing medical treatment. It is not always possible to avoid injections into the affected area, but you should inform the healthcare professional that you have lymphoedema or are at risk of lymphoedema and that they should try to avoid using the affected limb for non-emergencies. Similarly, you should avoid having blood pressure readings on the affected side.

- ***Swelling related to heat***

  People with lymphoedema sometimes experience more swelling in hot weather. This cannot be easily avoided, and the increased swelling will usually improve as the weather cools. However, you should avoid artificially hot situations such as saunas and steam rooms which may increase your swelling.

- ***Act quickly with signs of Cellulitis***

  If you develop signs of infection such as redness or rash, increased swelling, the area feels hot touch, or you feel generally unwell with signs of fever you should seek medical advice as soon as possible. If you develop symptoms out of hours you should telephone 111 if you are in any doubt and inform the operator if you have lymphoedema.

Please remember that good skin care is an essential component in the self-management of lymphoedema and when performed daily will quickly become a normal part of your daily routine. If you require any further assistance or guidance, please speak to your lymphoedema therapist or GP who will be able to advise you regarding best management for any specific concerns.

Top Tip #19: Put a sticky note on the skin care guidance page, for ease of reference.

12

HEALTHY LIFESTYLE

"Movement is one of the best things you can do to keep your lymphoedema under control."

—Rebecca Elwell,
Msc Lymphoedema

Now, I know what you might be thinking......*let's just skip this chapter and move on.....I don't need a lecture on what I should eat and how often I should move.* I totally get it, believe me. Stay with me though. Remember this book is from a fellow comrade in arms (or legs) with lymphoedema and I have to deliver on the title of the book and explain *How to Live Better with Lymphoedema*.

Let me be straight with you here. I am, by no means, a healthy eating fitness freak who spends hours in the gym and counts the calories of every meal.

I am going to be completely honest about my lifestyle and not make any false claims or lecture you on what the textbook tells us. I will say though, that at my very first appointment in 2012 with Professor Mortimer and Dr Gordon at St George's Hospital, I was told to lose some weight and exercise more. Sound familiar? An extract from their follow-up letter stated: *"General information given on lymphoedema and advice on the need to exercise, keep active whilst continuing compression and elevation of the leg at rest and at night."* Of course, I tried to justify that the extra weight and high BMI was due to my large and extremely heavy leg, but they didn't buy it, and so I became committed to lose some weight and get active.

Top Tip #20: Calculate and monitor your own Body Mass Index (BMI) using the calculator on the NHS Live Well website. The considered healthy BMI is between 18.5 and 24.9. *https://www.nhs.uk/live-well/healthy-weight/bmi-calculator/*

As this subject is one of the four cornerstones of lymphoedema management, I *had* to include it in my book or I wouldn't be very popular with my medical experts! I don't know about you, but the words diet and exercise can actually demotivate me. I don't want to diet. When I think of the word diet, it screams no fat, no carbs, no sugar, no alcohol, less meat, more fruit, more veg, more seeds and pulses, daily weighing, urgh! When I think of the word exercise, it shouts regime, discipline, all weathers, daily routine, double uurrgghh!

However, I find that I am more accepting of this concept if I refer to it as healthy eating and movement, or in short, a healthy lifestyle. Yep, I can work with that! Let me take this opportunity to share with you my experiences and challenges in trying to maintain a healthy lifestyle.

Let's face it, many of us like food that is not necessarily good for us. A real problem can be how much of it and how frequently we eat it. Healthy eating as I see it, is about balance and moderation, which I occasionally find difficult to achieve, as I will explain shortly.

It is widely reported that a healthy lifestyle involves good nutrition and physical activity, which can help you to achieve a healthy weight and maintain it. Maintaining it, however, isn't always easy.

In addition to helping you to manage your lymphoedema, a healthy lifestyle and maintaining a healthy weight can reduce the risk of developing Type II diabetes, heart disease and some cancers, which again is well publicised.

At every appointment with my therapist, one of the first things they do is measure my height and weight to calculate my Body Mass Index (BMI). This usually tells me that I am overweight, thanks! What did surprise me, perhaps somewhat naively, is that when I have put on a bit of weight, my leg measurements increase on both legs. Naturally, I notice any weight increase myself when my trousers get a bit tighter around the waist, or I see more than one chin in the mirror, but I hadn't realised that my legs would get bigger, which isn't great when having lymphoedema.

I now understand that a larger waistline can exert pressure on the groin area, which interrupts the lymphatic drainage to the inguinal lymph nodes. This is of particular relevance to me as I have been diagnosed with ilioinguinal sclerosis. (Ilioinguinal nerve is in the groin area and sclerosis being the stiffening of a tissue or anatomical feature, usually caused by the replacement of the normal organ-specific tissue with connective tissue.) I have just finished eating a satsuma, so all is good then, right? Wrong! Last night I scoffed several bags of 99cal crisps accompanied by some red wine, whilst watching a documentary about the talented actor and comedian, Robin Williams, who sadly took his own life, aged 63, during his battle with the progressive Lewy Body Disease.

Although I have been told by William Repicci from LE&RN that lymphoedema can be life-threatening, I believe it to be rare, so I should look on the bright side and cherish each day. It's up to me to look after myself by staying fit and healthy and wine and crisps won't help.

2020 and 2021 will be remembered mainly for the global Covid-19 pandemic, that claimed millions of lives around the world. It will also be remembered for the lengthy periods of lockdown which affected so many people in different ways. For my family, thankfully, just our daily routine was disrupted. Some people were able to continue their jobs in their usual workplaces and some had to adapt by working from home. Some were motivated to use the time effectively by improving their homes and gardens. Some watched programmes on TV about improving their homes and gardens. Some took the opportunity to go out for walks and get out of the house. Some people were either unable to, too afraid to, or didn't want to leave their house. Some people got fitter, whilst others got fatter.

The dreadfully stark and sad daily briefings from the Government were a constant reminder of the fragility of life, yet the British public did what the British public do and soldiered on. My family was inspired by 100-year-old Captain Sir Tom Moore, who walked 100 circuits of his garden and raised a colossal £38.9million for four charities. His much-loved saying "*Tomorrow will be a good day*" will be remembered by many. In addition to Captain Tom, the likeable, energetic and ridiculously fit body coach, Joe Wicks MBE, motivated millions of people to participate in his daily online workouts, raising £580,000 for NHS charities.

Both Captain Tom and Joe Wicks were motivated to exercise to raise money for charity. Selfishly, I am motivated to exercise to improve my health and, hopefully, to prevent my lymphoedema getting worse by me being overweight. Equally, I don't want to cause any life-threatening illnesses due to being obese and dying in the prime of my life. I have a lot to live for.

The only person who can actually influence my healthy lifestyle is me. I have to want to look after myself, eat the right foods and increase the amount of movement I do every single day. I look back at the last few months and can honestly say that I've sat for far too long at my desk writing my book and website and have not moved as much as I should have. Not good enough, Hazledine!

Top Tip #21: Set an alarm on your phone for every 30 minutes throughout the day as a reminder to get up and move about. Alternatively, invest in a Fitbit which monitors your movement automatically.

Lockdown restrictions prevented me from playing golf with my friends, or even alone which I find very therapeutic. However, I used the time to go for daily walks around our local area, or on longer country walks with a friend, when allowed. I have played netball with my daughter in the garden and tennis, of sorts, hitting the ball to each other in the local park. We even got the frisbee out last summer. In January 2021, I dusted off my mountain bike and started riding it around our town initially, then gradually further afield around local villages. When permitted, I rode alongside a friend for nearly 15 miles on and off road on a gloriously sunny day. I mostly cycled alone, with my mobile phone if required, and took in the wonderful scenic countryside and distant rolling North Downs. It gave me time to wind-down, clear my head and just, well, relax. Don't get me wrong, I wasn't racing about like I was in the Tour De France. In fact, quite the opposite, slow and steady meant I could increase the distance I cycled. Because cycling is non-weight bearing and non-impacting, it is really good for my leg and also my mental wellbeing. This doesn't feel like exercise to me, just a pleasure to de-stress. I highly recommend it.

Swimming is also enjoyable and gets every muscle moving. I'm not a strong swimmer and often use the resistance of the water to stride from one side of the pool to the other, which my therapist told me is extremely beneficial for those with lower limb lymphoedema. I don't have to wear my stocking in the pool either, which is incredibly liberating. In our garage at home, we have several cardio machines, weights and dumbbells for us all to use. The cross-trainer is probably my favourite machine, as it isn't an impact exercise like running. Just 20 minutes whilst watching the news on the TV or tablet is sufficient to get my heart rate up and my muscles pumping. I combine this with doing the plank for one minute each day, which I am led to believe uses every muscle in your body. The main objective is to keep moving and not to stay sitting down for any length of time and if I do, to elevate my leg to assist the lymphatic drainage. The toughest thing for me is being disciplined to do something linked to exercise every single day, which is why I prefer the term movement. Movement is important to get the muscles pumping which helps the fluid flow around the lymphatic system. When I'm less active, my leg swells noticeably which is extremely frustrating. I have an easy weapon in my armoury to solve this. Get moving more often.

To help me create and sustain a routine, I wrote out a daily plan to balance working at the desk with movement breaks. For example, I allocate 30 minutes in the morning before I start work, to do the plank and cross-trainer. I break from work at 12pm and either go for a walk around the block or a cycle ride around the local area, for around 40 minutes, before putting the kettle on and preparing lunch for 1pm. When my daughter finishes school, we shoot some hoops (well she does, I mostly miss) which can take anything from 15-30 minutes. Yesterday, she even got me bouncing around on her trampoline and seeing who could go the highest on her swing. I find that I am more disciplined when I am working to a structure, or agenda. (I can hear my old work colleagues laughing at this.)

Writing this book has meant that my routine has temporarily gone to pot a bit, well a lot to be honest, so I have set my alarm on my phone to remind me to get up and move, which I will do right now before I talk about food.

Top Tip #22: Ask your lymphoedema therapist for information on the types of movement or light exercise that are particularly suitable for your personal circumstances.

I was intending to start this chapter with a section talking about healthy eating. As you can see, however, I have neatly swerved the subject to talk about movement instead. In our family, that's known as an HDT - Hazledine Diversionary Tactic. If I'm not keen on talking about a particular subject or answering a specific question, then I manoeuvre the conversation effortlessly to a new topic, which I have just demonstrated.

Food is fabulous and I love it all, except for broad beans, kidney beans and offal. Other than that, everything is fair game. Annoyingly, some of the foods I like aren't great for my waistline but what I have recognised, is if it's not in the cupboard it's not there to eat. We have changed our shopping habits for the better.

I usually have three healthy meals per day, including either reduced sugar muesli with semi-skimmed milk or poached eggs on wholemeal toast for breakfast; a sandwich and fruit for lunch; and a meat/fish dish with a selection of fresh veg and potatoes for dinner. However, I occasionally lose all sense of self-discipline and demonstrate a severe lack of understanding of the word 'moderation' and find myself bingeing on the bad stuff. The odd thing is, I can go for weeks without a chocolate bar or a packet of crisps, or even an alcoholic drink. Then BAM. If the mood takes me and I fancy a savoury snack of the potato variety, I will eat a 150g bag of Tyrrells Sea Salt & Cider Vinegar crisps, or a few of the smaller, normal sized bags of crisps that my daughter has for her packed lunch. The same thing with chocolate, nothing for months and then Easter arrived and I polished off a large chocolate egg and its contents. To help control my occasional urges for sweet treats Vicki boxed clever with her next order of Magnum ice creams and ordered ones the size of my thumb!

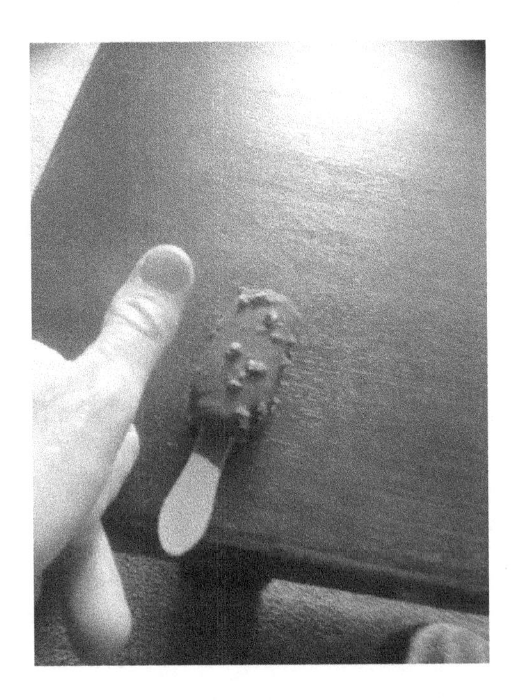

Portion Control – Bitesize Magnum Ice Cream

Top Tip #23: If you do fancy an unhealthy treat, limit the portion size or quantity to help you to maintain a healthy weight.

The only positive that I can take from this, is that I don't do this frequently enough for it to become a problem and I compensate by increasing the exercise, sorry, movement.

At just under 6' 4", I am of solid build with a bit of cushioning around the waist. My weight fluctuates between 17 and 17½ stone, although with much concerted effort prior to surgery in 2017 and again in 2019, I dropped to 16½ stone, so I know I can do it. The difficulty for me is sustaining it and I am my own worst enemy. To help me monitor my weight, a couple of years ago I produced a line graph on Excel where I record my weight on the first day of every month. The line graph clearly shows the trend upwards, downwards or static. It's an instant visual guide as to where I am. It may help you, perhaps.

Top Tip #24: Produce a line graph in Excel and record your weight every month. It's an instant visual guide on weight loss and gain.

The trick for me is to spot my weaknesses and try to avoid them.

The best example I can give you is this one, and please understand that I am sharing this with you for the greater good, just in case there is anyone else with lymphoedema who can relate to me and may benefit from my experiences.

If I'd had a stressful week at work, I would look forward to relaxing in front of the TV late on a Friday or Saturday night when the family had gone to bed, to catch up on the numerous episodes of Match of the Day that I had recorded. Not too bad so far. That is until I set up a selection of cheese and biscuits and a bottle of red wine, before pressing play and waiting for Gary Lineker to start the proceedings.

The trouble was (and I say was) this had become a bit of a habit, a routine that I hadn't set out in my original agenda. Once or twice a month, I would catch-up with the Premier League's finest accompanied by a cheese board and wine. In January 2021, I turned 50 and decided to take action and regain control. I deleted all the episodes backed up on the Sky Planner and cancelled the series link to prevent further enticement. Apart from the standard medium Cheddar and Red Leicester that my daughter likes, we don't buy any cheese that may lead me back to the dark side, such as Brie, Roquefort, Stilton, Dolcelatte and Boursin, to name a few. In addition, I now go to bed at the same time as my wife. I know! It's ground-breaking stuff, isn't it? The temptation for the 5 S's (Soccer, Stilton, Shiraz and Savoury Snacks) has been removed from my routine and deleted from the agenda. I spotted my weakness, took corrective action and sticking to the new discipline is now a strength.

Top Tip #25: Identify your weak spots, eg: certain times of day or triggers when you are more likely to eat unhealthy snacks or foods and change the routine. Fill that time with another distraction or swap the snack for something that is less bad for you.

There are two useful books listed on Amazon that stand out for me. One called "Lymphedema and Lipedema Nutrition Guide: foods, vitamins, minerals and supplements" dated April 2016 and written by a collaboration of authors including Chuck Ehrlich, Emily Iker and Karen Louise Herbst. Current UK price £10.44 reduced from £12.95 excluding delivery charges.

The other book is called "The Complete Lymphedema Management and Nutrition Guide: Empowering Strategies, Supporting Recipes and Therapeutic Exercises" dated September 2019 and written by Jean Lamantia and Ann Dimenna. Current price £18.95 excluding delivery charges.

As you can see by the spelling of Lymphedema, both books are written in America. While writing this chapter, I ordered the first book mentioned above from 2016, as it focuses more on food and nutrition and the free view pages showcase the content of the book very well. 24 hours later the book was delivered. I'm sure that I will glean many nuggets of valuable information that will benefit my life, making the £15 an excellent investment. I do hope that you are thinking the same about my book so far. There are other books available, so do check all publications listed on Amazon and other book retailers.

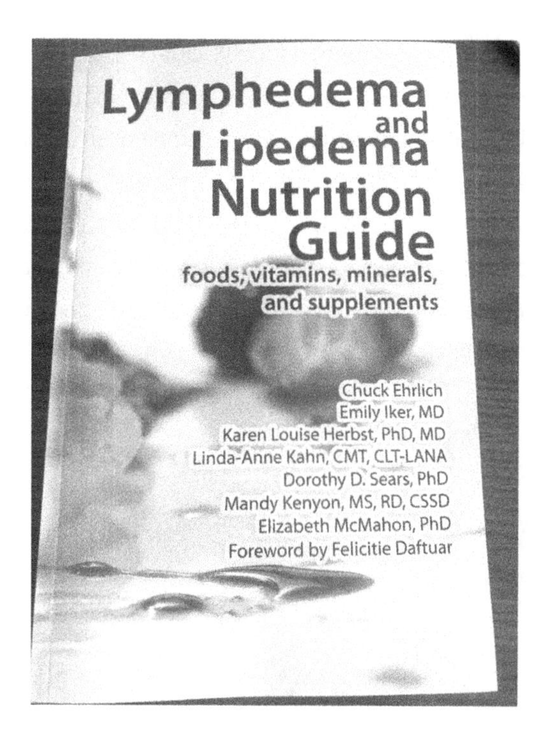

Lymphedema & Lipedema Nutrition Guide - Amazon

The advice from the NHS website *www.nhs.uk/live-well/eat-well* is very useful and well worth a read. It includes a clear message to eat less saturated fat, sugar and salt. Consuming too much of these increases the risk of developing heart disease, stroke, obesity and tooth decay.

Only I can make a difference as to how I live my life and I think the Covid-19 pandemic combined with becoming 50, has opened my eyes to really looking after myself.

Right, I've been sitting at my desk for far too long now. It's now 5.08pm and my daughter, Jasmine, is waiting for me to play netball and go on the swing with her. So now I'm going to practice what I preach and move.

I'm back and got beaten at netball 10-8 by Jasmine, but at least it's getting closer and not the thrashing I usually receive!

I wrote earlier about Captain Tom and Joe Wicks, who became national motivators, and I am very pleased to introduce you to another one. During the British Lymphology Society *#EveryBodyCan* campaign in 2021, Lymphoedema Advance Nurse Specialist, Rebecca Elwell, became an online sensation by producing and appearing in numerous videos on various social media channels. Rebecca provides motivational advice about movement and maintaining a healthy lifestyle. I am thrilled that she is sharing her expertise in this chapter.

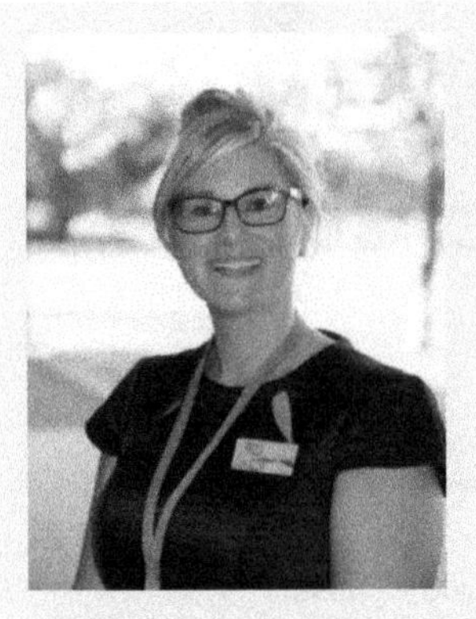

Rebecca Elwell Msc Lymphoedema

Macmillan Lymphoedema ANP and Team Leader, BLS Trustee

I am delighted and feel very honoured to be involved with your book Matt, which I know is going to be a great success.

The importance of a healthy lifestyle for lymphoedema patients

The British Lymphology Society's 'EveryBodyCan' campaign sets out to highlight importance of movement in both the management and prevention of lymphoedema. Unlike the heart, the lymphatic system doesn't have a pump, so we need to help it along. When we move our bodies, our muscles pump and we breathe deeper. These actions increase the flow of lymph around the body.

This prevents or reduces any swelling, as well as helping our body get rid of bacteria and other unwanted substances.

It's known that movement is good for our heart and lungs. It can help to strengthen our joints and bones, relieve pain and reduce fatigue; it's also good for our mental health. However not everyone knows it's great for our lymphatic health too.

A healthy lymphatic system is key to our overall health because the lymphatic system helps defend the body against illness and keeps our body fluids in balance. When the lymphatic system isn't working properly, fluid builds up in your tissues, which causes swelling (lymphoedema) as well as other health problems.

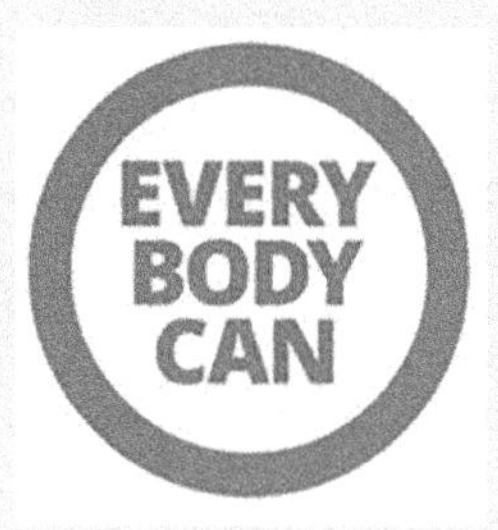

The EveryBodyCan campaign aims to find your Secret Weapon that encourages you to move. This maybe something in the home, e.g. the kettle as it makes you stand up to make a drink or it may be a gate on a field you lean on to feed a horse after a walk, or it may be something that helps you get really active like a skipping rope or walking boots. Walking fairly briskly is great for stimulating lymphatic function but you can also keep yourself active and healthy by doing more 'everyday' activities in the home or garden and being more aware of avoiding long periods of sitting still. When you are sitting it is important to position your swollen areas well, e.g. if your legs are swollen elevate them on a stool or if your arm is swollen rest it on a couple of pillows. And remember to go to bed to sleep at night wherever possible rather than falling asleep in a chair?

Movements should be carried out regularly throughout the day and throughout the week. They should be activities that we build in to do without thought like cleaning our teeth or washing our face rather than thinking of it as exercise which requires motivation in order to undertake it. If exercise could be prescribed it would be the number one prescribed medication in the UK and remember lots of activities are FREE. We ALL need to take responsibility to self-medicate with activity and find something that we can do regularly to get us and keep us moving.

It's really important if we find mobilising difficult to look at alternate ways of getting more active this may be chair based exercises, there is an NHS video available at: https://www.youtube.com/watch?v=E-JgZygWBKaE and multiple videos on YouTube for chair based yoga, Tai Chi and many other low-impact activities. Some local areas will provide funding to help with attendance at gyms and there are community clubs ask your GP for more information or check out the resources at your local library.

Remember any movement is beneficial no matter how small, anything which involves moving, stretching and breathing more deeply is good. Movement is one of the best things you can do to keep your lymphoedema under control. Most forms of exercise are safe, even weightlifting but it is important to discuss any plans for being more active with a lymphoedema practitioner or other knowledgeable professional, especially if you've been inactive for a while.

Don't forget if you have been prescribed a compression garment, always wear it when being active and make sure it is a good fit. Breathe deeply to encourage better circulation of blood and lymph. Build up gradually. If you notice swelling becomes worse, stop the activity until the swelling goes back down. You can restart but take it a bit slower and easier. For more information visit: https://www.thebls.com/pages/patient-resources

But it is not only movement which is important in our general health, our bodies requires fuel.

Although there are no specific diets recommended for lymphoedema (except in very rare cases). In order to live well, healthy eating is really important. Eating well can prevent heart disease, high blood pressure and diabetes as well as help weight loss. Being over-weight can make your swelling worse and can restrict your activity which again leads to an increase in swelling.

It is important to eat a rainbow of coloured fruits and vegetables daily up to 10 different types a day is recommended by the government but 5 as a minimum along with lean meat or fish or non meat based products for vegetarians or vegans e.g. beans/pulses. Carbohydrates should be wholegrain or high fibre versions if possible, e.g. brown rice or pasta and dairy products lower fat/sugar options whenever possible. Remember not all fats are bad cut down on saturated fats and replace them with unsaturated fats e.g. oily fish, nuts. Always try to avoid processed food, cut down on salt and sugar intake as well as alcohol. For more information visit: https://www.nhs.uk/live-well/eat-well/eight-tips-for-healthy-eating/

Drinking at least 6-8 glasses of water a day is recommended (water, no added sugar cordial or lower fat milk) and will not increase swelling.

Wherever possible you should try to stop smoking as this can affect your blood circulation, if you need help see your GP and for more information go to: https://www.nhs.uk/better-health/quit-smoking/

A healthy lifestyle has a positive effect on our mental well-being, when we feel positive we feel strong and more able to cope. We suffer less fatigue and are able to manage pain more effectively; this means living with a long-term chronic condition like lymphoedema can feel less like an uphill struggle. This, combined with the support of your local lymphoedema service (if you are lucky enough to have one) can give you the best control of your swelling, with their advice regarding on-going compression options and alternative treatments where necessary combined with you taking the lead and reducing your risk of infection, eating well and moving more it is possible to live well with lymphoedema.

Thank you, Rebecca, for your authoritative information and very helpful guidance. I will certainly aim to comply, especially with this next element which I need to constantly remind myself to do. Drink more water! It's been an hour since I put a pint of water (with a Vitamin C supplement in it) on my desk. So far, I've not even taken a sip! Oh, my alarm has just gone off to remind me to move! Oh, too much to think about all of a sudden; drink water, get up and move. I better follow my own advice!

Top Tip #26: When watching TV, stand up and do some stretches every time the adverts come on, or if you find it difficult to stand, stretch out your legs and rotate your ankles in both directions.

A large sip, a walk around the garden and 10 squats later and I'm back to the desk. Rebecca and the NHS website advise drinking 6-8 glasses of ***fluid*** every day. Fluid, not just water. Time to find out more. On clicking on the link "drink plenty of fluids" The Eatwell Guide says 6-8 glasses of fluid can include water, lower fat milk, sugar-free drinks, including tea and coffee. That's a relief, as I'm not really a water kind of guy. I drink lots of squash, no added sugar or sugar-free, naturally, plus the occasional Coke Zero or Pepsi Max, both sugar-free, so I am probably close to the target. How big is the glass though? Personally, I aim to drink at least four pints of squash per day.

There is an excellent product that helped me during very busy times at the office, when I would forget to drink water, or 'didn't have time' to refresh my glass. It is a 750ml water beaker with equally spaced time markers, which act as a reminder to drink a certain amount every hour from 8am to 6pm. Around lunchtime, I'd have to refill it for the afternoon's consumption, which meant I had to walk down and then back up a couple of flights of stairs to the kitchen, so that killed two birds with one stone. This product caught on in the office and at home, so I thought it may be of benefit to you. They are available in selected retailers probably for less money, but for ease, type "Water beakers with time markers" into Amazon search, to have a look at the range of products.

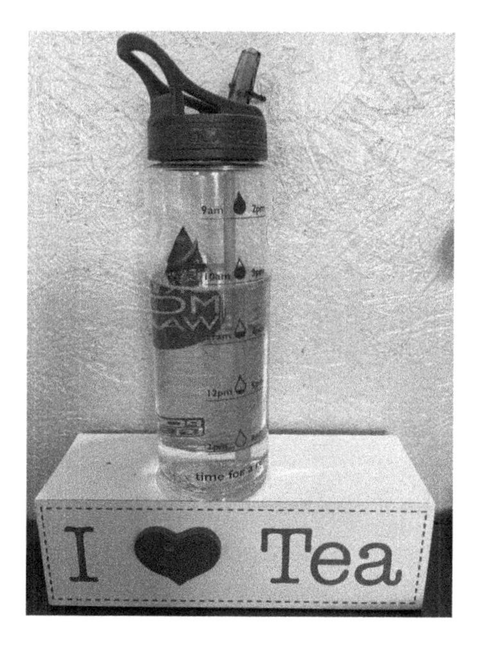

750ml water beaker with time markers

> **Top Tip #27: Purchase a water beaker with time markers on, to motivate you to drink the right amount of water or fluid per day.**

Just for the avoidance of any doubt, alcohol does not qualify towards your daily target of fluid intake.

Alcohol does contain more calories than I realised, which is counteractive to weight loss goals if not consumed in moderation. I am sure this is common knowledge, but as a reminder, the NHS Live Well website states that a standard 175ml glass of 12% wine contains 133 calories and a pint of 5% strength beer contains 239 calories. As we all know by now, the guide is an average of 2,500 calories per day for a man to maintain a healthy body weight and 2,000 calories per day for a woman. Therefore, if I drink 2 glasses of wine every night, I am using up 10.64% of my daily calorie count on alcohol, not including the odd packet of crisps that may accompany the wine from time to time, or previously the cheese. During the Covid-19 lockdown during 2020/21, I think it's fair to say that alcohol consumption increased in many households across the UK, ours included.

Top Tip #28: Assign 3 days of the week when you do not drink alcohol, preferably together, eg: Monday to Wednesday.

Top Tip #29: Limit alcohol consumption on Thursday and Sunday as, typically, weekend consumption is higher.

Writing this chapter has certainly reminded me to be more aware of what I eat and drink, and how much. Perhaps writing this book has presented me with the opportunity to shed any current bad habits, routines and lifestyle choices and make the concerted effort to return to a healthier lifestyle. I think this has been the kick up the backside that I needed.

13

DECONGESTIVE LYMPHATIC THERAPY (DLT), MULTI-LAYER LYMPHOEDEMA BANDAGING (MLLB) & COMPRESSION WRAP SYSTEMS

"It is personally quite satisfying as a lymphoedema specialist to witness the positive difference that we can make both physically and perhaps more importantly, mentally, to our patients."

—PATRYK GAWRYSIAK (MSC PHYSIOTHERAPY), CSP

In this chapter, we explain how an intensive course of Decongestive Lymphatic Therapy (DLT) can significantly reduce the volume of your affected limb or area in a matter of just three weeks. This therapy can be positively life-changing by reducing volume, and therefore the weight of the limb, and reshaping the limb back to as close as it should be.

Approaching eight months after getting lymphoedema in my left leg, I had my very first appointment with Professor Peter Mortimer and Dr Kristiana Gordon at the Lymphoedema Clinic in St George's Hospital, London. This was thanks to Mark Pearson, a therapist at St George's. I had found Mark on the internet when searching for a local therapist and was receiving treatment from him at his private practice towards the end of 2011. Mark told me about Professor Mortimer and that I *absolutely* had to see him, as he was (and still is) *the* 'go to' expert in the world of lymphoedema. At that time, I would have taken *any* help and advice from *any* expert and bought *any* product that claimed to treat lymphoedema. Some might say I was clutching at every possible straw to try and get my 'normal' life back again.

My supportive GP referred me to St George's Hospital and soon afterwards the letter arrived confirming my first appointment on 8th February 2012. I felt as though I had seen a glimmer of light at the end of this terribly dark and unfathomably long tunnel. Vicki and I were genuinely excited about meeting Professor Mortimer and we were full of high expectations and, more importantly, hope. The appointment went exceptionally well. I was thoroughly examined and listened to attentively, before a plan of action was discussed and agreed. Wow! At last, progress. We left St George's absolutely buzzing.

Under the care of the lymphoedema therapists at Hospice in the Weald and now, with additional advice and treatment plan from Professor Mortimer, Dr Gordon and the St George's team, we would soon get this lymphoedema in check, wouldn't we?

A few days later, we received the follow-up letter from St George's confirming the key points discussed and a plan of action for my GP, therapist and I, to implement. This is an extract from the letter for some relevant background information.

"St George's Hospital NHS Trust: Letter from Dr K Gordon, after seeing Prof Mortimer for the first time. Secondary infection in operation site, needing an inside drain for 2 months. Suffered a severe episode of cellulitis in June 2011, causing sudden swelling which hasn't gone back to normal since.

Lymphoscintigraphy shows a block below the left knee. Under the care of Hospice in the Weald and private MLD with Mark Pearson. Examination revealed lymphoedema in left leg from ankle to groin and there is fibrous scar tissue and lymph nodes palpable in the left groin. Evidence of mild folliculitis, otherwise he has a healthy skin and subcutaneous tissue.

Our first and most likely differential diagnosis is ilioinguinal sclerosis*, *although the rare possibility of a lymphatic malformation was also entertained by Prof Mortimer. General information given on lymphoedema and advice on the need to exercise, keep active whilst continuing compression and elevation of the leg at rest and at night. He would also benefit from decongestive therapy and might benefit from wraps over compression and continue with MLD."*

***NB**: After our third meeting in October 2012, Prof Mortimer's follow-up letter stated *"His lymphoedema is due to obstruction at the level of the left inguinal glands. I suspect this was originally caused by ilioinguinal nodal sclerosis, but I cannot be sure."*

These 177 precise and succinct words in his first letter to me contained a brief background, results of the examination, a diagnosis, guidance on the key elements of self-management and specific advice to both GP and therapist, that I would *'benefit from decongestive therapy and wraps over compression, while continuing with MLD'.* That all sounded extremely encouraging and positive, so let's get cracking and book this in, I thought. But what was 'decongestive therapy'? Had Professor Mortimer explained this and we'd missed it, or had we forgotten what was said in all the excitement? This chapter gave me the opportunity to ask an expert to explain what DLT is.

I have experienced DLT and Multi-Layer Lymphoedema Bandaging (MLLB) countless times over the past 10 years. This compression therapy has always been very effective for me, producing a notable reduction in volume when comparing before and after photos, or measurements. The significant reduction in volume gave me the confidence that the size and shape of my leg could be controlled, which really lifted my spirits.

The tremendous challenge I still face today is maintaining the reduced size, as my lower leg, in particular, is prone to gradually rebounding several weeks after treatment concludes. However, when my leg was smaller and lighter, I had more energy and less pain and discomfort, which in turn improved my mental wellbeing and kept my chin up. In the back of my mind, though, I always knew that if my leg did get too big, a three-week session of DLT and MLLB would do the trick and bring the volume back down again. This therapy has been such a vital part of my lymphoedema management regime.

To find out more, who better to ask than the Specialist Physiotherapist in Lymphoedema and Team Leader from St George's Hospital, Patryk Gawrysiak. Before I share some of my personal experiences, Patryk will explain more about these types of compression therapies, including how and when they are most effective.

Patryk is responsible for the Team of Lymphoedema Therapists, most of whom have provided me with DLT and MLLB treatment as both an outpatient and inpatient at St George's Hospital since February 2012.

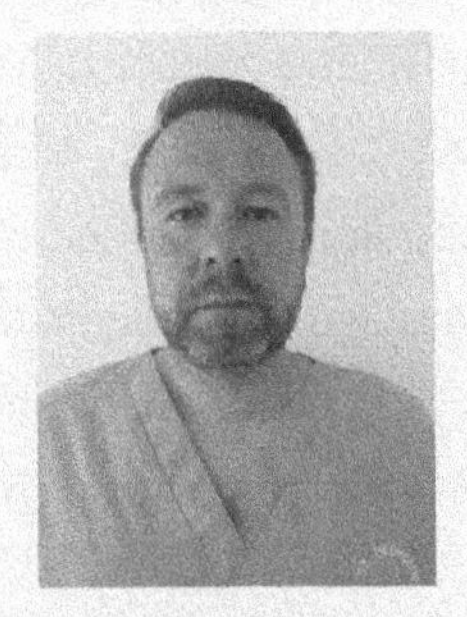

Patrick Gawrysiak
Lymphoedema Team Leader/Specialist Physiotherapist in Lymphoedema (MSc Physiotherapy), CSP

Was it really that long ago? Time has marched on and I am pleased to see that Matt is in a much better place than when I first met him at our lymphoedema clinic. It is personally quite satisfying as a lymphoedema specialist to witness the positive difference that we can make both physically and perhaps more importantly, mentally, to our patients. I am delighted to feature in Matt's book and hopefully demonstrate to many other people with lymphoedema, that with the right treatment, from qualified lymphoedema therapists, you can return to some degree of a normal life.

At St George's Hospital Lymphoedema Clinic, the journey begins with the initial consultation meeting and getting a good understanding of the patient's circumstances, background and personal needs. Typically, the starting point with any new patient is to discuss the cornerstones of self-management in addition to the range of treatments and compression aids that we, as therapists, can help them with. The priority for us is to reduce the limb volume as much as possible using a variety of methods, before arranging the correctly sized compression garments and educating the patient to apply the self-management disciplines daily. This usually starts with Decongestive Lymphatic Therapy or DLT. So, what is DLT?

The NHS state on their website that Decongestive Lymphatic Therapy (DLT) is the recommended treatment for lymphoedema. DLT is not a cure for lymphoedema, but it can help control the symptoms. Although it takes time and effort, the treatment can be used to bring lymphoedema under control.

There are 4 components to DLT:

- ***Compression Bandages***

  The specialist application of various layers of individual bandages, applying compression to the affected area which helps move lymph fluid out of the affected limb and minimise further build-up

- ***Skin Care***

  To keep the skin in good condition and reduce the risk of infection (see Chapter 9)

- ***Exercise***

  To use muscles in the affected limb to improve lymph drainage and compliment the DLT therapy

- ***Gentle form of massage techniques***

  Known as Manual Lymphatic Drainage (see Chapter 12) which stimulates the flow of fluid in the lymphatic system and reduces swelling

DLT is an intensive phase of therapy, during which you may receive daily treatment for several weeks to help reduce the volume of the affected limb or body part. This is followed by a second phase of treatment called the maintenance phase. You will be encouraged to take over your care using simple self-massage techniques such as Simple Lymphatic Drainage (SLD) (see chapters 14 and 15), in addition to wearing compression garments, continuing to exercise and complying with the skin care regimen. This phase of treatment aims to maintain the reduced size of the affected limb, as a result of DLT, with regular reviews every few months to check how your treatment is progressing. The second phase is largely dependent on the compliance of the patient in continuing to perform their duties in the self-management treatment progress, or potentially the affected limb will rebound to the size prior to the Decongestive Lymphatic Therapy (or even go beyond it), which would be a huge step backwards for the patient.

In this chapter we focus on Multi-Layer Compression Bandaging and Compression Wrap Systems, often called Velcro wraps.

The lymphatic system has no central pump to move the fluid to the lymph glands, unlike the heart pumping blood circulation around the body. Instead, the lymphatic system uses the contracting effect of surrounding muscles to move the fluid, which is why exercise or movement is important.

Water exercises are considered one of the best forms of exercise due to the additional pressure the water offers (swimming, aquarobics, aqua-cycling). Compression bandages or garments, such as sleeves, gloves, stockings or tights fitted over affected limbs act as a counterforce to muscles. This stimulates more effective lymph drainage. The combination of compression and exercise encourages the fluid to move out of the affected limb. Compression garments should also be applied after a massage session to prevent the fluid accumulating in the affected limb again. Velcro wraps may also be used instead of bandages or compression garments, as they are designed for self-management and can be easier to apply yourself.

Multi-Layer Lymphoedema Bandaging (MLLB)

The aim of Multi-Layer Lymphoedema Bandaging (MLLB) is to help the lymph fluid to drain and prevent it from building up, or pooling in a certain area or limb, typically, but not exclusive to, the arm or leg. MLLB can also assist the affected body part return to their normal shape. We provide MLLB as part of Decongestive Lymphatic Therapy (DLT), which will usually involve daily bandaging for a 3-week period. MLLB can be complimented by receiving Manual Lymphatic Drainage (MLD) to improve the flow of fluid to the lymph nodes and therefore assisting volume reduction.

MLLB should only be done by a fully trained and qualified lymphoedema therapist, as the bandages are applied in a specific way. MLLB may not work effectively if the bandages are uneven, too loose or too tight, which may cause discomfort and could further damage the delicate lymphatics. If done incorrectly, it could result in increased swelling or an uneven build-up of swelling. The objective is to reduce the volume of the affected limb and try to regain the proper shape of the limb, as close as possible. Before starting the MLLB therapy, it is important to measure the circumference of the limb at numerous equal points, which enables us to calculate the limb volume. It is incredibly rewarding and motivational for both the patient and the therapist to compare the limb volume and measurements from before and after the MLLB therapy. We often see reductions in limb volume of up to 40%, which makes the 3 weeks of intensive therapy completely worthwhile.

There are various methods of MLLB and different bandages available from specialist lymphoedema suppliers. We start multilayer lymphoedema bandaging by washing the leg/arm, applying an emollient adequate to the skin condition to moisturise the limb, before covering the complete limb with a lightweight elasticated tubular bandage. The product we use at St George's Hospital is called Comfifast but there are others that can be used. It is comfortable against the skin and protects it and can be easily cut to the appropriate length of the limb. We roll the end back at the foot or hand, so we can apply a very thin, light bandage to the toes or fingers, which is done in a very specific way to reduce swelling in this area.

When resting, elevation of the limb is important during MLLB therapy as fluid can drain downwards and if the bandages are not correctly applied, the fingers or toes could increase in size and become uncomfortable. Once this part has been completed, we roll back the tubular bandage to fully cover foot, leaving quite a bit spare to fold back later as a cover. We also leave the toes open depending on the patient's preference. We then apply several layers of soft synthetic wool or foam, ensuring additional padding behind the knee/elbow and across the top of the ankle/wrist, as these areas need extra protection. Again, these bandages are applied in a certain way to provide an even layer of padding and comfort. In some cases, we will use special foam e.g. "spaghetti" foam to give additional padding and protection to areas such as the knee pit, or across the top of the ankle. This is to prevent pressure sores or ulcers. We now move onto applying short stretch bandages, starting at the foot/hand and working up the limb, in a figure of eight or spiral motion, until the top of the thigh or armpit area. It is very important that these bandages are applied at a consistent level of stretch and compression to encourage the fluid the drain in the correct direction and back into the main lymphatic system. Getting the application of these bandages wrong could easily result in further damage to the lymphatics, or create an ulcer, or cause numbness, if too tight. Alternatively, if too loose, the bandages will soon slip down and will not provide the level of compression required to successfully drain the lymph in the correct direction.

We finish the MLLB process by applying a further tubular bandage carefully unrolling it over the short-stretch bandages and folding over at the foot and hand for protection and comfort. This is mainly to protect the short stretch bandages from becoming misplaced by rubbing against clothes. The tubular bandage is soft and enables clothes to easily slide over it. As you will expect, the size of the limb has increased significantly with this multilayer bandaging and we warn our patients in advance to bring loose fitting clothes to wear after MLLB therapy.

Then the patient usually returns home, encouraged to do gentle exercise and regular movement, as MLLB is most successful when the muscles are moving against the compression bandages and helping to pump the fluid to the lymph nodes. At their next visit to clinic, we ask the patient to help to remove the bandages to save time, before washing the whole limb with a soap substitute and patting it dry. It is then at the discretion of the individual therapist whether they provide Manual Lymphatic Drainage massage, or use an electric automated compression pump, which simulates MLD massage (see chapter 17), usually for between 30-45 minutes. Once this has been completed, the Multi-Layer Lymphoedema Bandaging process starts all over again. This process is usually done daily, or every other day, for a 3-week period or longer. The patient is usually unable to drive due to the size and rigidity of the limb, so we advise a family member or friend brings them to each appointment.

At the very last MLLB session, we measure the limb and calculate the volume, which is usually and pleasingly much less than before treatment began. Prior to this point, usually at the end of week 2 or week before the end of DLT, we will measure for new compression garments to be produced, using our expertise to forecast what the final measurements are likely to be by the end of week 3. Delivery of the new compression garment is received in time for the final day of MLLB therapy, with the objective being to maintain the reduced size of the limb. The intensive therapy should provide a significant and noticeable reduction, but it is important that the patient continues with the self-management plan, to help to maintain the size, because if neglected, the volume could rebound quickly if not properly managed.

Compression Wrap Systems

Because Decongestive Lymphatic Therapy and, in particular, Multi-Layer Lymphoedema Bandaging is so intensive, time consuming and costly, it is usually available on the NHS once per year to each patient. Therefore, to help the patient to maintain the limb volume, easily and conveniently at home, it is common practice to advise the use of Compression Wrap Systems, sometimes referred to as Velcro Wraps. There are many versions of this product available from a number of the specialist lymphoedema suppliers and manufacturers. It is worth asking your therapist or GP if you can get the wraps on prescription, as they can be quite costly. Albeit, if you have to purchase them yourself, the wrap systems provide a simple solution to help you to manage your lymphoedema, especially in times of periodic swelling, perhaps due to standing on your feet for long periods of time, for example.

Compression Wraps come in several sections to cater for individual needs. Wraps for legs come in 3 parts for the foot, lower leg and upper leg including the knee support. Some manufacturers also provide a separate knee section. Wraps for the arm usually come in 2 sections for the hand/wrist and the whole arm (above the wrist). Antimicrobial Liners are available to wear underneath the wrap systems, for comfort. In some cases, it is advised not to wear wraps on top of your usual compression garments, so please check with your therapist for advice about your condition and requirements.

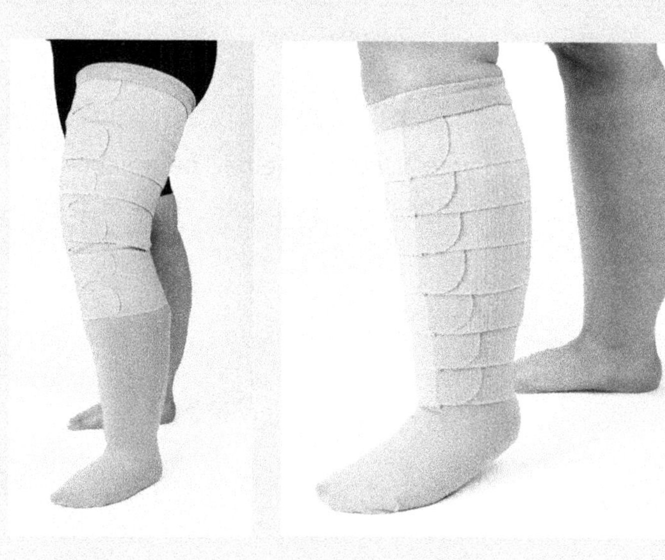

Compression Wrap System - Upper Leg   Compression Wrap System - Lower Leg

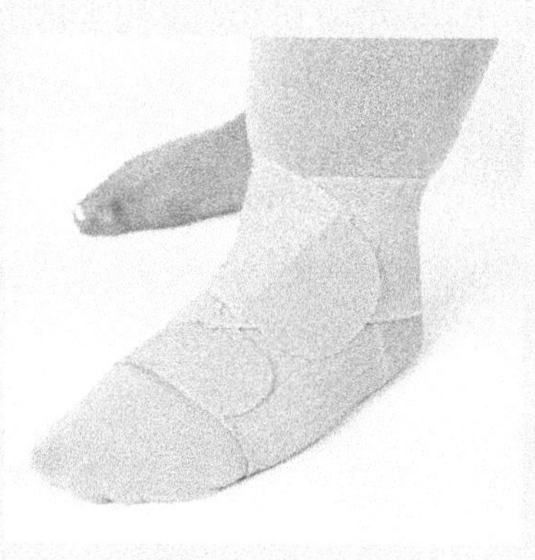

Compression Wrap System - Foot

Some Wrap systems are available in 2 levels of compression strength. For example, the brand that we have used for years at St George's is the Haddenham easywrap range. For legs they offer a light compression at 20-30 mmHg and a strong compression at 30-40 mmHG.

There are many different combinations of sizes available, and as always, it is advised to seek expert advice and help from your therapist, to ensure you order the most suitable product for personal circumstances.

Top Tip #30: Talk to your Lymphoedema Therapist or GP about arranging Decongestive Lymphatic Therapy (DLT), if you haven't already.

Thank you, Patryk. My first three-week course of DLT and MLLB was in April 2012 with my therapist at Hospice in the Weald.

Thankfully, this proved to be extremely successful. I experienced a reduction of 2,054ml of fluid (more than a 2-litre bottle of Coke Zero!) and a reduction in volume from 47% to 31% bigger than my right leg. I couldn't begin to tell you how excited I was to get to just over 31%. It was actually 30.5% but the figure had to be rounded up, regardless of my protestations to record it as 30%. This amazing result put a huge spring in my step and I genuinely thought we had found the solution to my problem. Frustratingly, though, it wasn't long before my leg started to rebound in size and at my next appointment, just six-months later, my leg was back up to 41% in volume at the start of the following MLLB session.

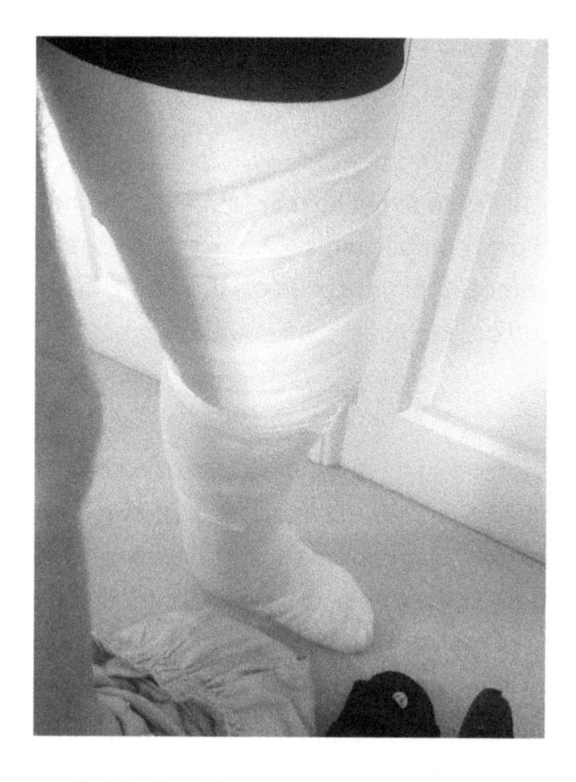

Matt's leg in Multi-Layer Lymphoedema Bandaging

Unfortunately, mid-way through the three-week treatment period in October 2012, we noticed that my leg was breaking out in white-headed spots at the hair follicle and many had begun to bleed. My therapist had no choice but to stop the MLLB treatment immediately as I had folliculitis, which is when hair follicles become inflamed, usually caused by a bacterial or fungal infection. The last thing she wanted to do was to continue the bandaging and risk further infection and inflammation. I started taking Flucloxacillin to prevent infection. I was advised to keep the skin clean and apply Dermol 500 Lotion, and to wear a class 2 compression stocking (instead of class 4S) to prevent further irritation until the skin healed.

The English weather can be very unpredictable as we know, and we experienced a scorching heat wave during another three-week DLT and MLLB session. No matter how hard I tried to keep my leg cool, it was a struggle under 4 layers of heavy thick bandages. We kept a very close eye on the possible reappearance of folliculitis, that's for sure.

Top Tip #31: Try to avoid having MLLB during hot weather to try and prevent folliculitis. Check the long-range weather forecast for your area on the Met Office website *www.metoffice,gov.uk*.

I had several successful MLLB treatments, resulting in a typical reduction in volume from 49% to 34%. My therapist and I would see a consistent gradual rebounding with the volume almost returning to the pre-treatment measurements. As a possible solution to break this cycle, my therapist proposed the idea of having two treatments back-to-back, over a six-week period, to really try and reduce the volume. The results were no different, with a reduction from 47% to 34% and then plateauing for the remaining few weeks of treatment. Although I was very satisfied with the reduction to 34%, unfortunately, this wasn't a long-term solution for me personally. Therefore, we needed a new plan.

Earlier in this chapter, Patryk explained the MLLB process perfectly. This method was used by the therapists at St George's Hospital when they treated me as an outpatient and also as an inpatient, when I had liposuction surgery (see Chapter 20).

The occasions that I had daily MLLB as an outpatient of St George's are my most memorable. The hospital is two hours' travelling time from my home, via a combination of train, tube and foot. I can tell you that my inhibitions about having lymphoedema went right out of the window then! Imagine the scene, a tall lump of a man with an enormously bandaged leg, walking up and down the steps at London Bridge Station, shuffling from side to side dragging this huge elephant leg along the underground platform and down the bustling Tooting Broadway. Now, I know anything goes in Cosmopolitan

London, but this was really pushing my boundaries of acceptability! Still, it was good exercise for me and got the lymphatics pumping.

Compression Wrap Systems

After many attempts of MLLB, I am resigned to the rollercoaster ride of downs and ups in leg measurements and quick, but unsustainable, volume reductions.

In my armoury of compression garments and aids at home, I have the easy-wrap compression wrap system from Haddenham Healthcare. I use the wrap system when my leg shows signs of increasing in size, which it still does from time to time, even after two different types of surgery.

To identify any notable change in leg size, I measure the circumference at four different points of my left leg, first thing in the morning, on the first day of every month. I record them on an Excel spreadsheet and line graph which helps me to spot trends at a glance. The four measurements are taken at the same points each time: just above my ankle; mid-calf; knee; and upper thigh. When I see a noticeable increase in the line graph, that is the time that I use the compression wrap system to boost the compression and try to reduce the size. In between times, the tightness of my trousers is an excellent guide too, of course. The chart works for me and may be something that could help you?

> Top Tip #32: Measure your limb monthly and record on an Excel line graph. If you see any increase in size, use a compression wrap system to try and reduce the volume. However, if you experience a constant increase in size, please contact your lymphoedema therapist for advice.

I seem to have more of an issue with the size of my calf now, than my thigh, especially after a long cycle ride or 18 holes of golf. I elevate both legs whenever I sit down to work, read a book or watch TV. For years I have used a high foot stool on wheels, to elevate my leg under my desk. However, my calf is up and down in size, like the Nutty Professor.

Top Tip #33: If you work at a desk for long periods, invest in a comfortable foot stool on wheels, that is the right height to elevate your leg, comfortably, under your desk.

The compression wraps are easy to put on, with robust yet soft material straps that fix around my leg, attaching to the other side of the garment with Velcro pads. This means that I can adjust the level of compression I need very quickly, so if the straps are too tight, it takes seconds to alter them to a more comfortable level. Now, the product information leaflet says that the wrap system can be worn under clothing, but that just isn't practical for me under suit trousers. I use them as and when I need to control the size and try and reduce ad-hoc swelling. This is a better compromise than giving up golf or cycling!

Top Tip #34: Ask your therapist or GP to prescribe appropriately sized Compression Wrap System to use when you experience increased swelling.

14

LYMPHATIC DRAINAGE TECHNIQUES AND KINESIOLOGY TAPE

"Any person who is seeking treatment for lymphoedema must be sure that a therapist is trained to provide Decongestive Lymphatic Therapy (DLT)"

—Carol Ellis MSc, BSc,
PGCert, FHEA. Chair of MLD^UK

There are many references to Manual Lymphatic Drainage (MLD) in this book, as it is one of the four well-known cornerstones to effective management of lymphoedema:

- Skin Care
- Compression

- Healthy Lifestyle & Exercise
- Lymphatic Drainage

In this chapter we focus on the fourth one, Lymphatic Drainage including MLD and Self Lymphatic Drainage (SLD). We also look at a relatively new therapy called Reflexology Lymphatic Drainage (RLD). In addition to these variations of specialist massaging techniques for people with lymphoedema, we investigate the benefits of using Kinesiology Tape to assist lymph drainage.

The first hurdle to overcome, perhaps, is being physically and mentally comfortable in allowing someone else to see your body and touch your swollen limb(s). This can be embarrassing for some people, me included, initially, which I am happy to expand on.

After recovering from the first episode of cellulitis and kind of coming to terms with my lymphoedema, we decided to book a spa break at one of our favourite getaways. Vicki and I both booked to have a massage, but I wasn't ready to undress below the waist and reveal my hugely swollen stockinged left leg. In fact, I felt so embarrassed about my body, that I nearly cancelled the spa treatment altogether. Understanding my discomfort, Vicki suggested instead of a full body, I could just have a head, neck and shoulder massage and remain clothed from the waist down. I agreed, well, she is almost always right anyway. This massage had the same effect on me and managed to uncoil my tight shoulder muscles. I, sorry Vicki, found a workaround to enable me to continue enjoying the trip.

As a separate point, pre-lymphoedema I would relax in the sauna and steam room. With lymphoedema, this is now totally out of the question, as the extreme heat increases the swelling in my leg and is not recommended by the experts.

I am less self-conscious when having MLD because the therapist has seen countless embarrassed, nervous patients with swollen limbs. MLD is a treatment for a medical condition and not the same as having some pampering, although I do find MLD incredibly relaxing now I have overcome my own self-consciousness. MLD therapists have seen it all before and given the opportunity to have this treatment my instant answer is a resounding *"yes please"*.

I have had MLD from several therapists over the years and was surprised to find that some of them used different techniques. The first time I had MLD, the therapist used small massage strokes that were light and gentle, starting at the ankle and working up the leg. Another therapist used much firmer deeper strokes, almost like a sports massage. Some therapists begin by opening up the lymph channels in the abdomen and shoulder, gradually working down the body and others just open the channels around the waist and groin. I subsequently found out that there are different recognised techniques of MLD.

To explore further, I invited Carol Ellis, Chair of MLD^{UK} to explain about the history and various techniques, in addition to providing an overview of the organisation.

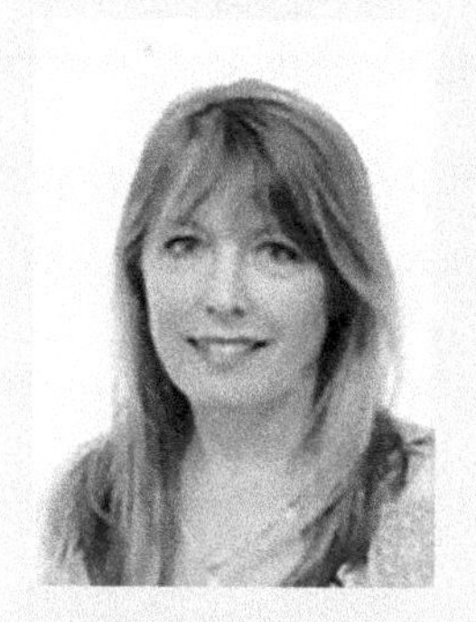

Carol Ellis MSc, BSc, PGCert, FHEA
Chair of MLD^{UK}

Further to a telephone conversation with Matt, during which he was telling me about his experience with lymphoedema, he told me about his aim to put a book together with relevant, reliable evidence- based information to make the journey easier for other lymphoedema patients. With contribution and feedback from MLD^{UK} committee, we have put together a chapter on the history and development of MLD, the different techniques, levels of training and how to access a suitably trained therapist.

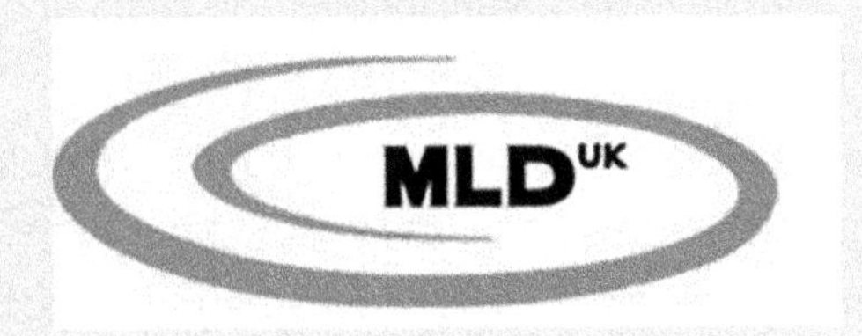

Introduction

Initially trained in Vodder method of Manual Lymphatic Drainage (MLD) in 2001, then the Le Duc method in 2009. I have work as a Lymphoedema Practitioner at a charity run cancer support centre since 2002, working with patients with secondary Lymphoedema. This role includes providing lectures/workshops on Lymphoedema in hospitals for healthcare professionals, and various cancer support groups, and charities like Breast Cancer Now 'Moving forward' education programme providing information on Lymphoedema for breast cancer patients.

I am also employed as a Senior Lecturer at ARU university, in the Faculty of Health, Education, Medicine, and Social Care lecturing in research skills for undergraduate students from various disciplines.

What is MLD

Manual Lymphatic Drainage (MLD) is more a skin treatment than a form of massage. It is a slow, gentle, low-pressure, rhythmic and repetitive technique which stretches and relaxes the skin, and varies the pressure, in order to increase the functioning of the lymphatic system. A range of specialised movements follow the direction of the lymphatic system, working from the neck down to the limbs. The gentle stretching techniques stimulate the contractions of the lymphatic vessels, helping to move the lymph forward, whilst pressure changes and circular movements of the skin cause more lymph to be formed from the fluid, protein and waste products present in the tissues (Foldi and Foldi, 2012). These techniques can help to reduce swelling, bruising, and inflammation, and may also reduce pain. According to Zuther and Norton (2018), it is the slow, repetitive movements of MLD affecting the autonomic nervous system which can both reduce pain and provide a calming, relaxing treatment.

History of MLD

MLD was first developed in France in the 1930's by the Danish Emil Vodder. Although his professional background is uncertain, he had an interest in skin, physiology and general health. His technique was originally designed to help a person suffering from sinusitis. Following this initial success, he expanded his technique to include all parts of the body. However, his attempts to market his technique were interrupted by war. A decade or so later, the Vodders created a clinic in Walchsee, Austria, which still exists in the care of the family who were taught by Emil Vodder. Around the same time, the Vodder technique was adopted by the Drs Michael and Ethel Foeldi, who established their clinic in highest Black Forest, for the treatment of the lymphatic system. Henri Leduc, a physiotherapist, and John Casley-Smith, a lymphologist, developed their own MLD techniques in the 1960s. The Leduc method was used in his clinics in Brussels and Paris, whilst the Casley-Smith technique was introduced to Australia though, like Vodder, they are now known worldwide. MLD is used extensively by the health services of the German-speaking countries and is acknowledged by many European lymphoedema clinics to be one of the four cornerstones of conservative management of lymphoedema, along with skin care, exercise and compression (Foldi, Foldi, 2012).

Benefits of MLD

A well-functioning lymphatic system is essential to health; waste substances and fluid are removed from the tissues and returned to the blood following some processing within the lymphatic system. There is also its contribution to immunity; circulating lymphocytes and scavenger cells deal with infection and abnormal particles in the lymph. In enhancing the function of the lymphatic system, MLD can improve the health of the individual; in some European countries, it is commonplace for people to seek regular MLD as a health maintenance measure. It can also be routinely prescribed before and after surgery, to accelerate healing and reduce pain. Bruising and swelling may be reduced and wounds heal more quickly. The same effects can be seen when MLD is used following injury. It has not gained the same popularity in the UK but is frequently advised after cosmetic surgery or liposuction for the reduction of lipoedema.

MLD's capacity to remove fluid and protein from the tissues can improve the swelling of puffy ankles or eyes, and relieve the fluid congestion of pregnancy, though the latter should always be done in consultation with the midwife.

Where lymphoedema is present, whether primary and due to an inherent abnormality of the system, or secondary to surgery or cancer treatment, MLD can be seen as a vital component of treatment. Combined with other essential interventions, it can improve the lives of people with lymphoedema. Similar gains might be made where MLD is used to treat oedema caused by venous insufficiency.

Lipoedema is thought to be an abnormality of fat, which results in proliferation of fat cells. It may be associated with inflammation; the affected tissue tends to be painful, bruises easily and might be oedematous. MLD can provide some comfort to people with lipoedema, as it is gentle, reduces swelling and might decrease pain, both through a neurological effect and the possible removal from the tissues of the chemical mediators of inflammation. It may be these effects which appear to reduce the discomfort of conditions such as chronic arthritis, and the reduction of inflammation which leads to an observed improvement in acne and other skin conditions.

As was noted by Emil Vodder, MLD can be effective in reducing chronic sinusitis. There are other specific health problems which may be amenable to treatment by MLD; it is always worth asking.

Different techniques of MLD

Although MLD techniques vary in the details of hand movements and treatment routines, they all adhere to the fundamental principles. MLD should not be painful, and only heavy in pressure where fibrosis is being softened or, in the case of some methods, where the emptying of lymph nodes is being encouraged.

At present, MLDuk accepts therapists who have been trained in the Vodder, Foeldi, Casley-Smith, Leduc or Belgrado techniques, the latter being the latest addition. Developed in Brussels, it is taught by the Lymphoedema Training Academy.

MLD qualifications

Any person who is seeking treatment for lymphoedema must be sure that a therapist is trained to provide Decongestive Lymphatic Therapy (DLT), also known as Complete Decongestive Therapy (CDT).

Some MLD therapists prefer not to treat lymphoedema, instead providing supportive treatment for other chronic health problems or post-operative care.

A therapist who is described as an aesthetician has completed Vodder training in treatment of the face and neck, but this does not include lymphoedema.

Training

MLD training involves a combination of theoretical and practical learning. The theoretical component may be delivered online but a large proportion of the tuition is of necessity a matter of demonstration, direct supervision and many hours of practice. It is believed that there is no substitute for the tacit knowledge which is gained through observation of the expert practitioner.

All MLD therapists will have studied the anatomy and physiology of the lymphatic system and its normal pathways and functions. They will know how to apply MLD to most areas of the body. Manual techniques are demonstrated, and practised extensively by students; all MLD schools insist on robust training. It is expected that therapists will be able to provide supportive therapy for a range of chronic health problems, and to reduce the swelling and bruising which can result from surgery or injury.

Those therapists who intend to treat lymphoedema will study the causes and effects of a malfunctioning lymphatic system. They will learn to use MLD to reduce oedema through using alternative pathways and maximising the function of any unaffected parts of the lymphatic system. They must be able to apply compression through bandaging or special garments, and to advise a client about exercise and skin care. Many clients will be attending an NHS lymphoedema clinic but the MLD therapist can be an additional source of support for self-management of the condition.

It is expected that all clients will be fully assessed before any therapy is given, and that the progress of a client be evaluated and recorded. These skills will be incorporated into any training.

Kinesiotape

Kinesiotape is a thin, adhesive tape which, although woven from cotton, is highly elastic. This is due to its specialised weave. Originally developed in Japan as a treatment for musculo-skeletal injuries, it was found that correctly applied tape can lift the superficial layers of the skin, whilst the whorls of the weave will cause movements which may mimic MLD. Extra training is required before an MLD therapist is competent to use Kinesiotape; this may be part of treatment where it is deemed appropriate.

How to find an MLD therapist in the UK

*Suitably trained therapists can be found through the Therapists section of the MLD*UK *website, www.mlduk.org.uk. Entering a postcode will show nearby therapists, both their location and their distance from the post-code. Also, whether a therapist is trained to provide DLT.*

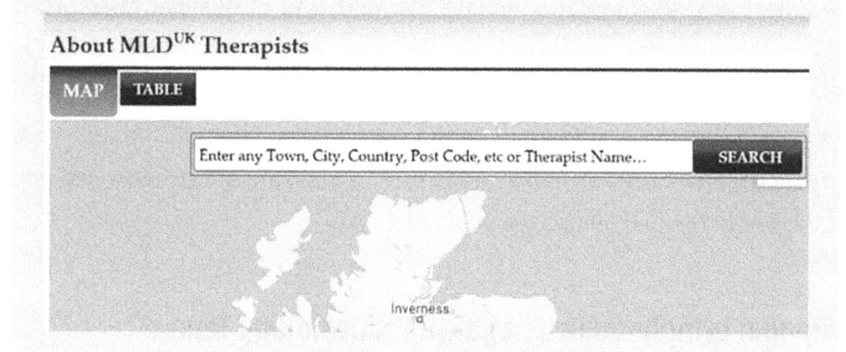

MLD UK Website Search Bar – Find a Therapist

To find your nearest qualified MLD therapist, visit www.mlduk.org.uk/therapists

Who are MLDUK?

*MLD*UK *was founded in 1995 as a voluntary regulatory body for MLD therapists. Its broad objectives are to ensure a high standard of MLD, and to support its membership. Applicants are required to provide evidence of appropriate training from one of the recognised schools. Then, because* *of advances in knowledge and the importance of maintaining skills, they must undertake a biennial update of both theory and practice. All members must carry adequate indemnity insurance and abide by the MLD^{UK} Code of Conduct and Professional Practice Guidelines.*

The current register of members, and other information about MLD^{UK} can be accessed by the general public and other healthcare professionals, through the website.

References are in Appendix IV

Thank you, Carol for taking the time to provide this information.

As discussed in Chapter 5, finding the right kind of qualified therapist is extremely important to ensure your lymphoedema is treated effectively. To help me find a local MLD therapist, I would use the MLD^{UK} website, as it only lists therapists who have undertaken training through the approved methods. This provides reassurance that those listed are experienced and qualified in Manual Lymphatic Drainage.

Manual Lymphatic Drainage with Kinesiology Tape

After my second liposuction surgery in 2019, I had several MLD sessions with a very experienced local lymphoedema therapist, Clare Anvar MSc. Clare applied Kinesiology Tape at the end of my therapy session. I spoke to Clare recently and she told me why Kinesiology Tape is used as a continuation of the MLD process.

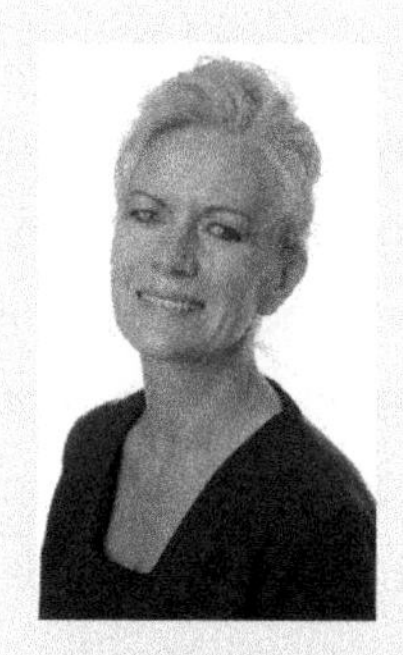

Clare Anvar BSc (Hons), MSc
MLD/Clinical Massage Specialist

Once MLD has cleared lymphatic pathways and stimulated drainage, Kinesiology taping is used to sustain these improvements. It is applied without stretch and positioned in strips from the nearest lymph nodes to the swollen area, so that the tapes wrinkle and straighten when the joints and limb are moved. The tape lifts the skin away from underlying structures, relieving tissue saturation and pressure, allowing the congested tissues to drain. This enhances the natural action of muscular contraction and moves lymph from areas it is not draining to places where it is. It keeps this process going between MLD sessions and can retrain the body to move lymph more effectively.

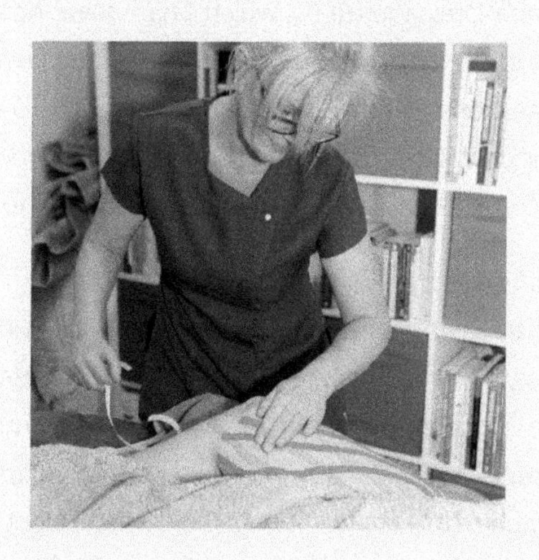

Clare Anvar MLD/Clinical Massage Specialist – Kinesiotaping

Self-Lymphatic Drainage

Self-Lymphatic Drainage (SLD) is an effective therapy that people with lymphoedema can do themselves as part of the self-management plan. I have also heard this referred to as Simple Lymphatic Drainage. For the purpose of this section, I will refer to it as SLD. This is covered in more depth by a professional lymphoedema therapist in the next chapter, so I won't pre-empt what's coming. I will just say at this point, that SLD is an effective method of drainage that we can all do in the comfort of our own home. It can be done in bed or watching TV in your chair (with your feet up) and doesn't take very long at all. As you would expect, there are countless videos on YouTube providing demonstrations on how to perform SLD. However, I would suggest asking your lymphoedema therapist to demonstrate and teach you SLD correctly to maximise the effectiveness. The last thing we'd want is to do ourselves any harm and further damage our lymphatics.

Reflexology Lymph Drainage

As I touched on in Chapter 5, when I searched on Google to find local lymphoedema therapists, two people on the search results provided a treatment called Reflexology Lymph Drainage (RLD), which I had never heard of. I have had reflexology many times with a local qualified therapist and friend, Jenny Hannon, but RLD was a new one on me. I spoke to Jenny about RLD whilst writing this chapter and coincidentally she had contacted Sally Kay to book a training course, so she could become a qualified RLD therapist, in addition to a Reflexologist.

I had to contact Sally to find out more and I have to say, what an amazing lady she is, with such enthusiasm to help people living with lymphoedema. Sally is a multi-award-winning reflexology practitioner, researcher, educator and author. She informed me she has developed RLD from first principles and through extensive clinical practice. This innovative approach to reflexology has attracted *national and international awards*, alongside widespread recognition. As a result of our conversation, I am delighted that Sally has agreed to write about her RLD therapy.

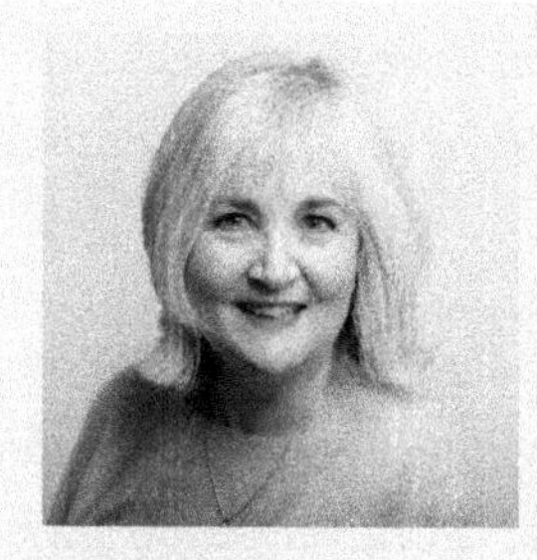

Sally Kay
Reflexology Practitioner, Author, Tutor & Researcher
Sally Kay Reflexology

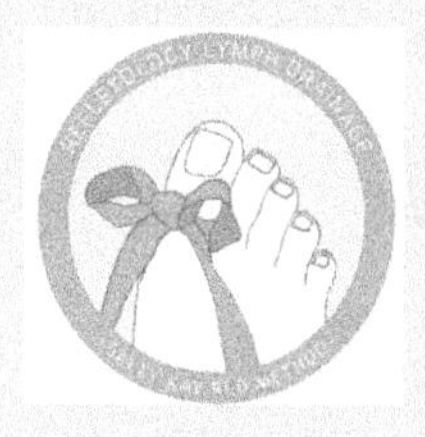

Reflexology is a relaxing, non-invasive complementary therapy, not an alternative one. It dates back thousands of years, historically practiced in ancient Chinese, Egyptian & Roman cultures to stay well. In the west we are more inclined to turn to it through ill-health and desperation, when things go wrong.

Reflexology is based on the theory that different organs and systems of the body are mapped on specific reflex areas of the feet (and hands). Typically, these reflexes are worked by the reflexologist with the aim to cause an effect in the body, in a relaxing therapeutic experience. It can be used alongside conventional medicine through each stage of life, including supporting couples with infertility at pre-conception, right through life, up to and including palliative care.

Reflexology Lymph Drainage RLD was first developed in 2010 while working in cancer care clinics, supporting patients at each step of the disease, from diagnosis, through their treatment to discharge or, end of life care.

Clinics were busy, typically seeing 20 – 30 patients a week, and sessions were time limited. Here, I was looking for innovative ways to adapt the reflexology to best help individuals.

This led to a problem specific, adaptive reflexology, and it proved to be extremely effective. Amongst other things, many of the patients were suffering with breast cancer related lymphoedema (BCRL) following their surgery and treatment. I have an advanced massage qualification but was not qualified to practice Manual Lymph Drainage massage (MLD), but I understood it. So, I adapted the reflexology to focus on the lymphatic reflex areas of the feet to reflect the principles of MLD.

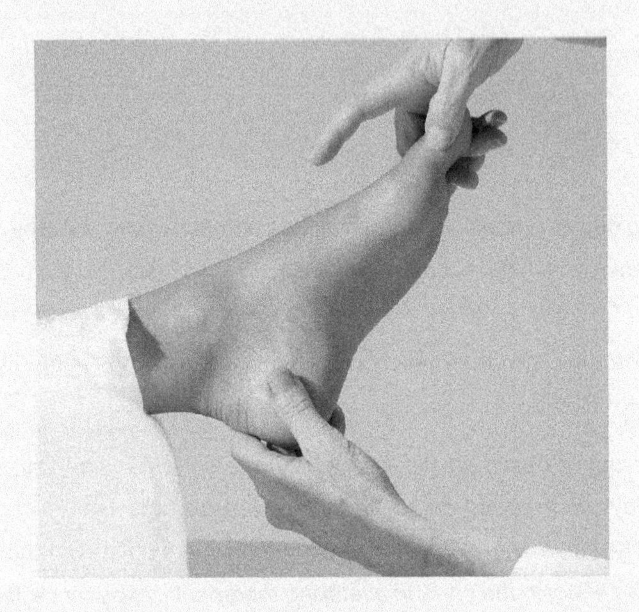

Sally Kay – Reflexology Lymph Drainage Therapy

Patients who received this could feel physiological sensations in the body, similar to their MLD experiences. Something was definitely happening! Clothing and jewellery became visibly loser, range of movement increased, and the results appeared to be cumulative and sustainable from one week to the next.

From my clinical experience I knew RLD was working and with the ability to measure these tangible results, I took a few small steps towards research. This approach has delivered consistent, phenomenal results and the facts and figures underline the impact my method of RLD has when these techniques are applied. There is such a positive ripple effect on quality of life when the swelling diminishes and lost self-confidence returns. To many people it is the gift of hope in a previously hopeless situation.

Bridging the gap between reflexology practice and proving its worth is notoriously difficult. I hope that my initial RLD research may form the cornerstone of future studies which will contribute to the understanding and integration of reflexology.

The statistically significant results of the RLD research (reference here), has gained recognition for this unique reflexology protocol worldwide, in the reflexology community and more recently in the lymphoedema community, Winner of 2019 National Lymphedema Network (USA) Award for Outstanding Contribution to Lymphology.

In the last decade I have taught RLD to reflexologists worldwide, they, in turn are successfully using the techniques to help their clients, and not just those with secondary lymphoedema. RLD is expanding to help clients with a wide and varied range of presenting conditions.

Modern day attitudes to health and wellbeing mean that we never stop learning whilst keeping an open mind to other therapies and innovations. Being a reflexologist is not a competition. Sharing and collaboration is, I believe the most effective way forward. After all it's only 80 years since the Vodders first began to explore and develop MLD.

For more information about RLD, please visit
www.reflexologylymphdrainage.co.uk

I would like to thank Carol Ellis, Clare Anvar and Sally Kay for their excellent insights into the various lymphatic therapies available to people living with lymphoedema. I really hope that you found this chapter interesting and that it has encouraged you to investigate MLD and RLD further, with a view to adding it to your lymphoedema management regime, if you haven't already done so.

15

LYMPHOFLUOROSCOPY GUIDED MANUAL LYMPHATIC DRAINAGE & SELF-LYMPHATIC DRAINAGE

"We now understand that in the right circumstances, you can drain the fluid down to nodes and skin that's draining well, rather than up!"

—Jane Wigg MSc, RGN Nurse Consultant, LymphVision

As we know, technology progresses at great pace and we have seen some incredible technological advances in medical science over the last few decades: smart phones, hybrid & electric cars and Artificial Intelligence for example. However, it sometimes appears as though these medical advances don't quite reach the lymphoedema sector, perhaps because the funding is not readily available.

I thought that lymphoscintigraphy was one of the most recent technological advances used for lymphoedema patients. However, in a national survey conducted by King's College Hospital and British Nuclear Medicine Society in Spring 2017, it was stated that lymphoscintigraphy has been performed in many centres in the UK since the 1950s. That's hardly recent.

Lymphoscintigraphy is a type of nuclear medicine imaging that provides special pictures of the lymphatic system, which transports fluid throughout your immune system. Lymphoscintigraphy is often used to identify the sentinel lymph node, or the first node to receive the lymph drainage from a tumour.

My first experience of having a lymphoscintigram was in June 2011, during my initial two weeks of hospitalisation from cellulitis. To be honest, I don't remember much about it, as I wasn't in a great place and in considerable pain at the time.

When I became an NHS patient of Professor Mortimer, he arranged for me to have a second lymphoscintigraphy scan at St George's Hospital, in July 2012, to assist him with my diagnosis. The results of the scan *"revealed reduced drainage on the left leg below the knee"*. This information was analysed along with the results of an MRI scan around the same time which *"revealed lymph nodes present on the left side which were more ill-defined compared to the right. There appeared to be lymph contained within the lymph nodes, supporting a diagnosis of ilioinguinal nodal sclerosis. There was also scarring in the left groin".*

In other words, I had issues with drainage above the knee, likely to have been caused by the cellulitis in 2011. In addition, there are drainage problems at the groin, very likely to have been caused by the surgery in 2007 for a suspected strangulated hernia, when the surgeon removed lymph nodes. No wonder my left leg struggles to drain lymph fluid properly!

In 2014, I experienced another scientific advancement which was used to investigate whether I was suitable for Lymphovenous Anastomosis (LVA) and/or Lymph Node Transfer (LNT) surgery. I had a CT scan and a Photodynamic Eye scan (PDE) at Broomfield Hospital in Essex. The PDE scan was fascinating to watch. Similar to a lymphoscintigram, dye was injected between my toes on both feet. I then had to walk around the hospital for a couple of hours to allow the dye to work its way up the lymphatic system. I was then reviewed by the surgeon, laying down, (me, not the surgeon) lights off, TV monitor on, a tube of lubricant gel and a hand held scanner. The surgeon placed the scanner on my foot and slowly moved it up the length of my leg.

On the monitor, I could clearly see the dye travelling along my lymphatic system up to the knee, where the clearly defined channels then stopped and turned into fabulously exploding fireworks, which he called star bursts. When he moved the scanner above the knee there was less of a prominent channel of dye, it was there, but not as obvious. Not that I'm an expert, but there was clearly an issue again at the groin which was the next area of blockage.

I then saw how the lymphatics should perform, when he switched the doppler to my right leg, showing a constant network of flowing streams all the way up my leg and up through the groin into the upper body. WOW! I much prefer looking at visuals to reading explanations and the visual clarity of this scan was amazing. I could see for myself where the issues were and, more importantly, so could the medical professionals. These results showed that LVA surgery was unsuitable for me (explained in Chapter 19) and we were able to proceed with LNT surgery planned for 2015.

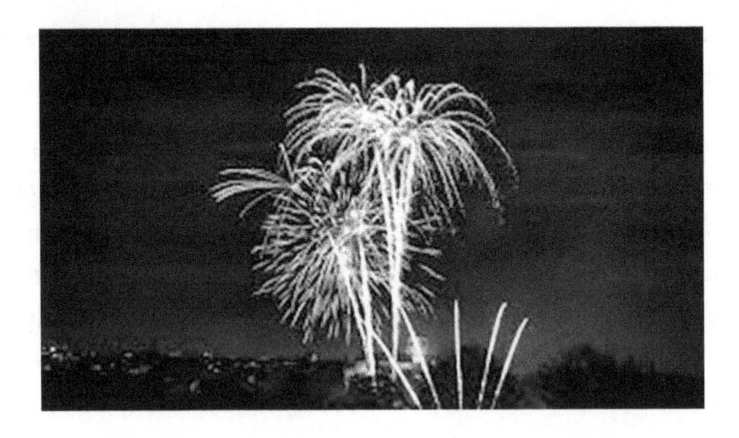

Fireworks representing the lymph flow and star bursting effect

More recently there has been some positive and exciting news to talk about. Lymphofluoroscopy Guided Manual Lymphatic Drainage.

I first met Jane Wigg at a British Lymphology Society (BLS) Conference in 2016, when I was a Trustee of the Lymphoedema Support Network (LSN). She explained her new business to me, which, I understand involves using a similar scanning technique to track the lymphatic flow and identify blockages. This mapping then provides valuable information to assist the therapist on where to focus and manipulate the flow of lymph fluid using Manual Lymphatic Drainage (MLD). That is a very simplistic explanation from my perspective as a patient. To provide a more professional explanation about Lymphofluoroscopy Guided MLD, I introduce you to Jane Wigg.

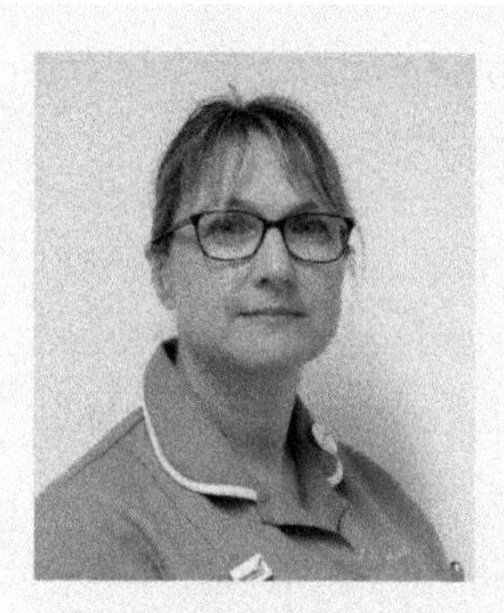

Jane Wigg MSc, RGN
Nurse consultant- LymphVision
Director/ Trainer Lymphoedema Training Academy
Lymphofluoroscopy guided MLD (FG-MLD®/ Fill & Flush)

I have met Matt a few times over the years at many of the lymphatic functions. I must have made enough of an impression for him to invite me to write a chapter in his book. We first met at quite a challenging time, where Fluoroscopy Guided Manual Lymphatic Drainage (FG-MLD®) and the use of ICG imaging, were being discussed as appropriate in the UK and we were causing quite a stir globally. This was generally due to lack of understanding and I'm pleased to say that lymphofluoroscopy mapping or ICG imaging is now relatively common practice in specialist centres. At LymphVision, we are quite unique in how we carry out this procedure, working as a detective and taking many hours to find the way your lymphatics are draining to assess how to help you best.

As the great Olivier Wendel Holmes Jr is known for saying, 'a mind that is stretched by a new experience can never go back to its old dimensions' and that's exactly what happened and continues to do so.

All great advancements begin with someone being a catalyst for change, and my thanks go to Professor Belgrado, who was a pioneer of Near Infrared Lymphofluoroscopy Imaging (NIRFLI). I had the privilege of being able to watch this trend with my work taking me to many international conferences. I knew we had to do something different, because 'nothing changes if nothing changes...' and so, change we did.

In 2014, Prof Belgrado trained our UK trainers and taught me NIRFLI. Here, we inject a very small amount of tracer called Indocyanine Green (ICG) just under the skin. This connects to proteins of the cells and flows through the skin to the lymphatics. Of course, sometimes the tracer doesn't get to the lymphatics, or it gets pushed back out of them and stays in the skin. This happens if they are blocked, removed, or absent. We use a special near infrared camera which reflects the light to a monitor to see different images and lymph move (I sold my holiday home in Bulgaria to buy mine!)

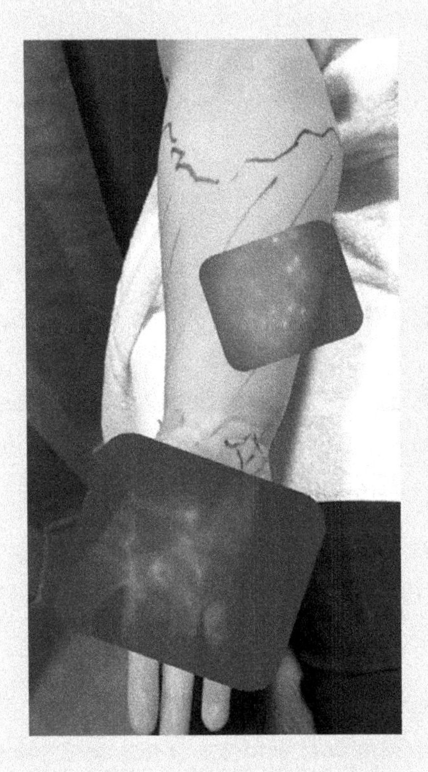

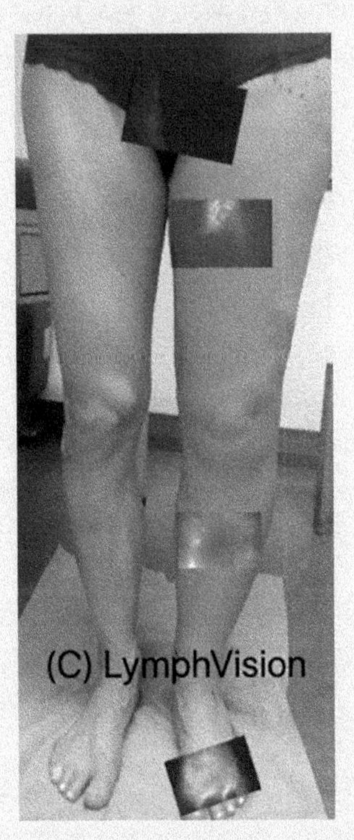

Examples of ICG imaging - arm and leg

Why Fluoroscopy Guided Manual Lymphatic Drainage? (FG-MLD®)

Well, why not? The very first time that I saw lymph moving, in real time, I knew that this had changed things forever. What we learnt from fluoroscopy, from the pioneering works of Professor Belgrado, is how many movements we need to move fluid and empty lymph nodes, if valves are working, where fluid is blocked, and where it is draining to. We learnt many other things also... we learnt that some of the drainage pathways that we have used for many years, are not always correct. We know that people have more chance of draining from one leg, across the abdomen and down the other leg, than they do draining to the axilla (armpit). We now understand that in the right circumstances, you can drain the fluid down to nodes and skin that's draining well, rather than up! The significance of these finding cannot be understated. They have empirically taught us things in recent years that we simply would not have believed when I started my career.

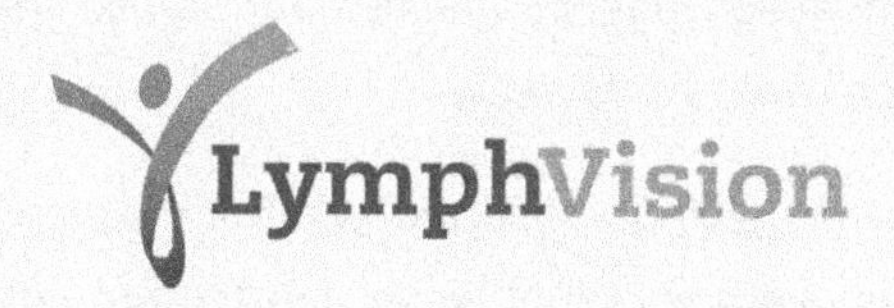

Through our clinic at LymphVision, we are able to offer lymphatic mapping to improve MLD drainage, screening to identify a lymphoedema at its earliest failure and pre-surgical mapping to identify areas to be avoided or any complications prior to reconstruction or breast cancer surgery. So, fluoroscopy is not only about mapping but what we have learnt has allowed for us to change our MLD technique and help more people.

Here are a few tips to help you with improving your outcomes.

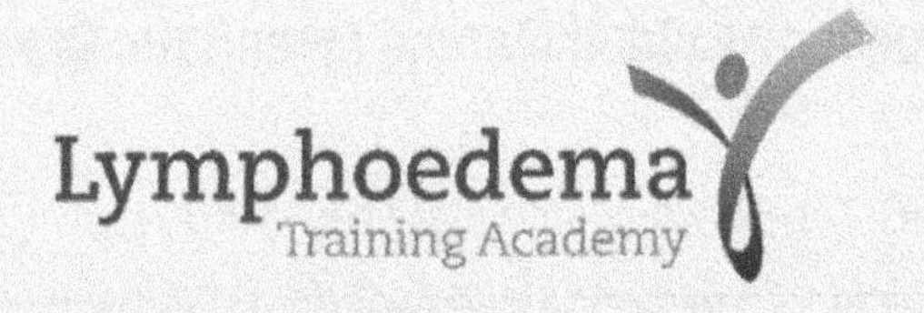

At Lymphoedema Training Academy we very much believe and teach that 'movement and drainage' is the key to improving your lymphoedema and this includes your Self Lymphatic Drainage (SLD). Of all of the things we need to do to maintain or reduce your lymphoedema, remember 'moving matters.'

- ***No drain, no gain.*** *Effective SLD does not have to be an overburden. However, for many they have been told that they need to carry it out daily for the rest of their lives. There is a different way. We recommend that you carry out SLD initially, many times a day, in order to reduce the fluid/filtration burden. This means that I would ask people to concentrate a period of time in their life where they can commit to this regime. I'd recommend that you carry out "little and often" because when we first see a therapist, 'no one came to be maintained', only improved.*

Imagine that you have a dripping tap, slowly filling a cup, and every day and night you remove a spoon of water, but the tap continues to drip every day, eventually overflowing. Now imagine that you have that same cup, but you repeatedly remove a spoon of fluid, many times a day for a few weeks; soon the cup is almost empty and you can now reduce how often you spoon it out. Controlling your lymphoedema with SLD is a bit like this. Commence five or more times a day for the first few weeks. Then you can reduce to three times day for a few weeks and hopefully at the end there will be a considerable amount of fluid loss. Of course, it's all very individual and you generally need to have the correct garments but the outcome should be that your lymphoedema will remain smaller, for longer.

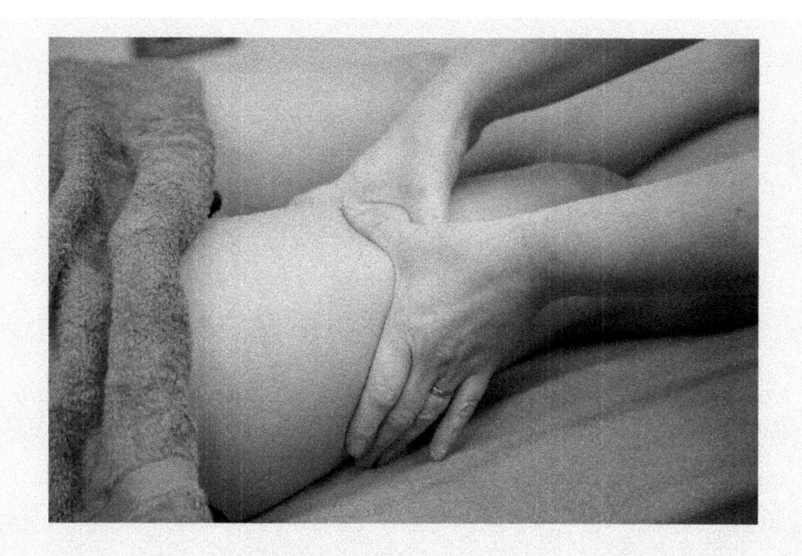

Example of Manual Lymphatic Drainage Therapy - thigh

- ***Empty your nodes.*** *You may know that as fluid returns back to the lymphatic system it will pass through the nodes. It makes sense then that the more that you empty the nodes the more the fluid can drain into them. Therefore, we recommend frequently emptying your lymph nodes. This is particularly important if you're not active because when your muscles pump, you push blood and fluid to the lymph nodes. If you are sitting, and inactive, lymph could pool in your legs or your arms. ICG imaging has demonstrated that four "good" squeezes to the appropriate area, are enough to empty nodes. This means that you can stop doing 10, we just thought a long time ago that this was a good number but has no evidence to support it!*
- *When doing FG-MLD® we now understand where to drain to and how to use your time more effectively. Many people with arm swelling, still drain to the armpit and many people with leg swelling still drain to the groin even though some nodes may be removed. Understanding if you have nodes working in those places means that you can save time draining to places that you don't need to.*

- *As a general principle, you can:*

    1. *'Flush', gently where there is no oedema, to clear the way*
    2. *Empty your nodes four times*
    3. *Work a little firmer on where the oedema is*
    4. *'Fill' the deeper lymphatics and,*
    5. *'Flush' it back to the nodes.*

Unfortunately, a short chapter cannot cover all the intricacies of the technique (even lymphoedema therapists require weeks of training!) but supporting videos can be found online and the pictures alongside will help.

Good luck, and remember 'No drain, no gain!'

Thank you for the excellent explanation Jane, which was obviously more comprehensive and succinct than my brief introduction summary. For more information about Lymphofluoroscopy Guided MLD, please visit *www.lymph-vision.com*

It is my intention to book an appointment with Jane to have a lymphofluoroscopy scan. I can then give the results to my local MLD therapist to assist her with maximising my lymph drainage.

Jane also sent me some images demonstrating how to empty lymph nodes using a LymphBall, that I could use as part of the SLD process for my leg, which may be of interest to you. I would imagine that the same principle applies to upper limb lymphoedema, by using the stress ball under the armpit and in the crease of the elbow joint.

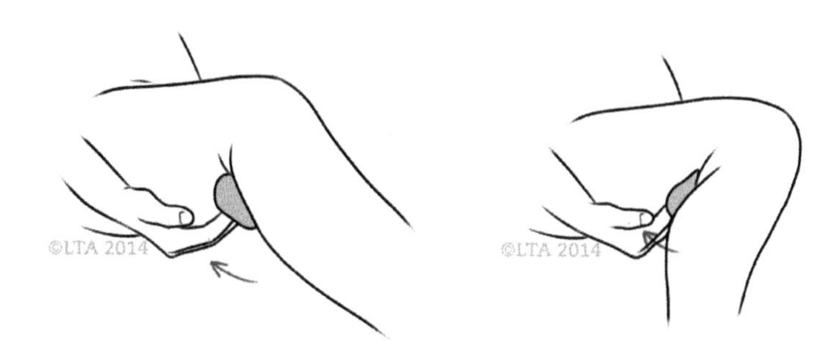

Above - LymphBall to empty popliteal lymph nodes right

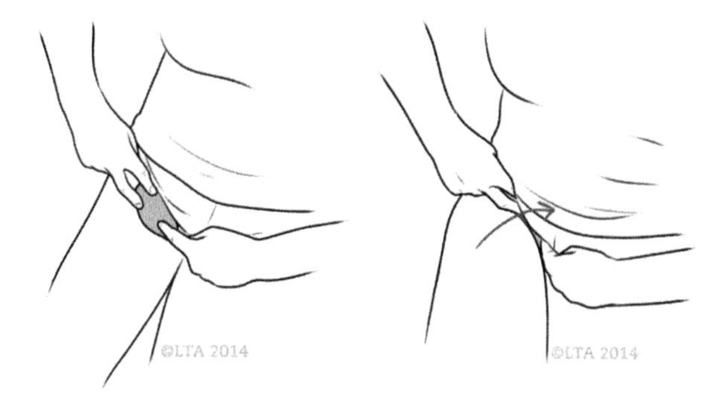

Above - LymphBall to empty inguinal lymph node right

16

CLOTHES & SHOES

"I've made over 1500 pairs of jeans and without a shadow of a doubt, the ones I have made for Matt are my most memorable commission."

—ELIZABETH RADCLIFFE, MASTER TAILOR. LEVI'S LOT 1

I do hope that this book is being read by men and women, as this chapter contains many solutions to help both sexes including children in sourcing 'normal' looking clothes and shoes for a lymphoedema-friendly wardrobe.

I, like so many people living with lymphoedema, face many different challenges, some of which can be very distressing. Firstly, one has to try to come to terms with the physical effect of the increased size of the limb(s) with swelling that is often difficult to reduce and maintain. Secondly, one has to cope with the effect that lymphoedema has on one's mental health and wellbeing, which can result in a loss of self-confidence and lack of self-esteem, brought on by changes in size and appearance. For me, and I understand I am not alone here, *one* of the biggest frustrations I had after being diagnosed with lymphoedema, was no longer being able to fit into my clothes or shoes. In addition to this, buying new replacements off-the-shelf was practically impossible.

I experienced tremendous despair that my new swollen leg and foot wouldn't fit into any of my trousers, jeans or shoes. I worked in the Financial Services profession, which meant weekdays the traditional work attire was a suit, or smart jacket and trousers. Outside of work, I was very much a smart pair of jeans and a polo shirt kind of guy. Over the years, I had accumulated a decent wardrobe of quality suits, trousers and jeans, plus a selection of shoes for all occasions. Without any exaggeration, all my trousers, jeans and shoes had become instantly redundant, except one pair of wide leg linen trousers which became my saviour at the time. Reading this back, it all sounds a bit dramatic and over the top, but I have always taken pride in my appearance and was comfortable in my own skin.

Lymphoedema had totally shattered my self-confidence in just a matter of weeks.

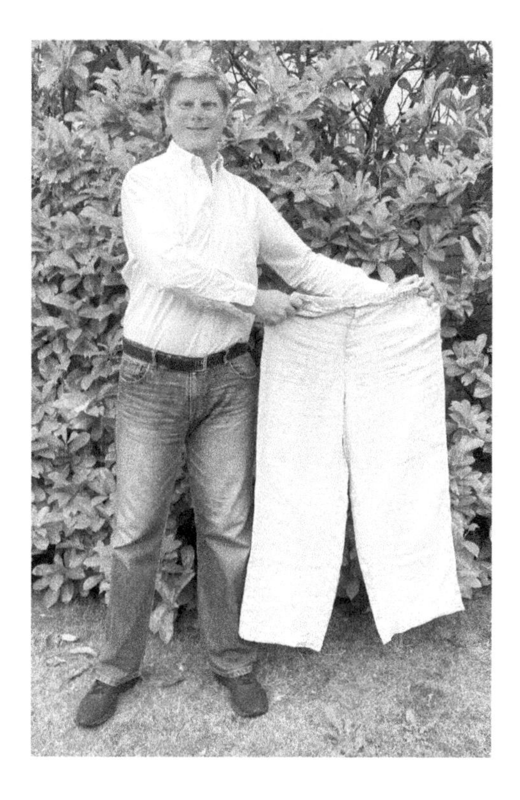

My 'go-to' pair of wide-legged linen trousers

Trousers

This may sound a bit self-centred and vain, but I enjoy looking smart and always remember my late grandfather saying to me that *"clothes maketh the man"* and to *"always shine your shoes so you can see your face in them"*. I Googled 'Big & Tall clothing' to try and find companies that sold affordable clothes and shoes. Disheartened, most of my purchases had to be returned. In some cases, I literally had to buy trousers that were humungous around the waist, to have any chance of getting my left leg in. They looked terrible and had the reverse effect of bringing me down further. When at the office though, I tried incredibly hard to hide my embarrassment and apply the Great British spirit of *"Carry on and smile through it"* as best as I could.

Then one day, like Worzel Gummidge, I put my 'solutions' head on and wondered how I could create a pair of trousers that fitted me perfectly for both legs and waist. In the first instance, I spoke to a local tailor, who, if I can be so bold, wasn't really interested in the challenge as I wanted each leg a slightly different width, the concept of which he couldn't grasp. Because it wasn't a typical order, I think he priced himself out of the job, at a cost of £650 for one pair of trousers and two pairs for £1,000.

Time for Plan B. I spoke to another local business called Zippystitch. I explained my situation with lymphoedema and told the seamstress my plan. Probably seeing my anguish, she accepted the challenge and quoted a much more realistic sum. Game On!

I went straight to my local Marks & Spencer's and purchased five pairs of sensibly priced, smart black trousers, probably around the £25-£30 mark each. I took them to Zippystitch for them to carry out the delicate operation and execute my cunning plan. As instructed, the tailor unpicked the seam of the inside leg of four pairs, from hem to crotch. Having measured the circumference of my left leg at the thigh, knee, calf and ankle, she used the fifth pair of trousers to cut the legs into long panels of material. She then sewed each panel into the inside left leg of each of the other four pairs. I hope I have explained that satisfactorily. As the sewn in panel was on the inside leg, it barely showed, especially as they were in black. The tailor charged me about £25 per pair and Hey Presto! I had four pairs of made-to-measure trousers for under £250. I was rather proud of my idea.

This was around mid-2012 and for me it was pretty life-changing stuff I can tell you. I was able to wear a smart jacket, shirt, perhaps a tie, with my new, smart, black trousers. I felt great and, being black, the trousers hid the size difference in my legs very well indeed.

After the first success in black, I tried to repeat the same exercise with a different colour, to mix up my wardrobe a bit. Not my best idea though, as the sewn in panel was more obviously visible in slate grey, as was the difference in the size of each leg. Black it is then!

These cut-and-shut trousers were my safe place for a couple of years before I had Lymph Node Transfer surgery in 2014 (more about that in Chapter 18). The outcome of the surgery wasn't as expected. After just a few months later, my leg volume had increased to the highest it had ever been, at 58% bigger than the right. Sadly, my 'go to' trousers were now redundant too and were put back in the 'spare' wardrobe just in case one day my leg would reduce in size again. I will explain my Plan C shortly as it's now time to talk about shoes.

Shoes

Of course, having perfectly fitted, smart made-to-measure trousers on a budget is one thing. Having the smart shoes to accompany them is another. It's perhaps no surprise that my choice in shoes has changed a bit since being encumbered with lymphoedema, as my life has changed substantially. As I have mentioned, for all of my professional working life I have worn suits, or jacket and trousers, with smart business shoes. After being diagnosed at the age of 40, I tried to find wider fit shoes that still looked appropriate with smart trousers. Not easy, but I found some, eventually.

In January 2021 I sold my business to focus on making a positive difference in the world of lymphoedema. Working from home means the daily wearing of smart trousers and shoes is no longer required, that is until Zoom calls are replaced by face-to-face meetings again.

I remember my first couple of visits with my therapist, Kelly Nickson, and me grumbling that I couldn't fit into any of my shoes because of my F'leg. She pointed to the windowsill, where there were several booklets from wide fit shoe companies, unlike anything I had purchased before. Well, I have to say that when my back was at its worst (I'll explain later), I came close to ordering a pair just for the pure 'comfy' factor. I didn't though, instead I found the brand Hotter online and ordered a pair from them. They were smart enough to wear with my new black 'cut-and-shut' M&S trousers, yet casual enough to wear with jeans. More importantly though, they were super comfortable and helped to make walking less painful. I have ordered since, this time smart brogues in both black and brown, which sit in the place where my previous shoes used to be.

Looking for a birthday gift for me, my lovely wife found a company online called iTailor that manufactures made-to-measure shoes, designed by you, using their innovative and interactive website. In addition to the bespoke shoes, there are many other styles for men and women to choose from. Sounds pricy right? Quite reasonable, actually, considering the lack of options available elsewhere. A typical pair of leather shoes cost £79 upwards and £149 upwards for custom made-to-measure. I ordered a pair to try them out and followed the instructions online to the letter, as measuring correctly when having lymphoedema is paramount. The first time I ordered a pair, I made the mistake of following the instructions a little too literally and took my measurements just wearing socks. On receiving delivery, the left shoe was tighter than the right shoe. Why? Because I hadn't taken account of the thickness of my compression stocking.

What I should have done, in hindsight, is keep my stocking and socks on to allow for a bit of wiggle room. The first pair got pushed to the back of the 'spare' wardrobe. Still, it was my fault, not iTailor's, so I tried again. This time I kept the stocking and socks on and added a couple of millimetres to the length and width, to allow for any daytime swelling. The results were awesome! I had a nice pair of smart shoes again that were extremely comfortable. I was so impressed with their service, I designed a couple more pairs in different styles, which were a bit more of a statement. If you do take the plunge to give this company a try, my advice is to accompany your order with an email, making it abundantly clear that you have lymphoedema and that your measurements are correct, even if they appear unusual to their shoemakers. It may also be useful to attach some photos of your feet as well. Good luck and have fun with it. Their website is *www.itailorshoes.com* and there is more to tell you about iTailor shortly.

Other shoe suppliers who provide a wider fit include: *www.hotter.com*, *www.widefitshoes.co.uk*, *www.cosyfeet.com*, *www.skechers.com* and *www.clarks.co.uk*.

My shoe collection is now looking much more like it used to, albeit with a few pairs of 'comfy' shoes than before, for good measure. But then again, I am 50.

Suits

The next step for me was to get a suit for occasions such as: business meetings; functions; weddings; and funerals. After lots of research and phone calls, I dismissed many expensive tailors commanding upwards of £1,500. I then heard about a company called Dress2Kill, a short walk from Waterloo East Station, London. I have since found out that they also have a shop in High Street, Andover, Hants. Catering for both men and women, they are an independent tailor with a difference. Their superb website is definitely worth a visit. Their range and prices are clearly listed, with the starting price of £525 for a two-piece suit, with additional pairs of trousers starting at £175. (Plan C.)

At my first appointment, I was made to feel comfortable and relaxed whilst I explained what lymphoedema is, before describing how I wanted the trousers to look and hang. Once measured, I browsed through several swatches to choose the material for my first ever made-to-measure suit. No surprise, it was black.

It really was a very enjoyable experience. A few weeks later I had my second appointment for the first fitting. I was thrilled with how the suit looked and more importantly, it fitted perfectly. What lymphoedema? Who would know? Great! I sat with a drink in their opulent waiting area, while the final tweaks were being made to the trousers. It wasn't too long before I was on my way, proudly carrying my new suit in its striking cover. I subsequently ordered an additional pair of trousers which took care of my Plan C, after sending my previous cut-and-shut trousers to the 'spare' wardrobe. I highly recommend their service and you can find out more on their website *www.dress2kill.com*.

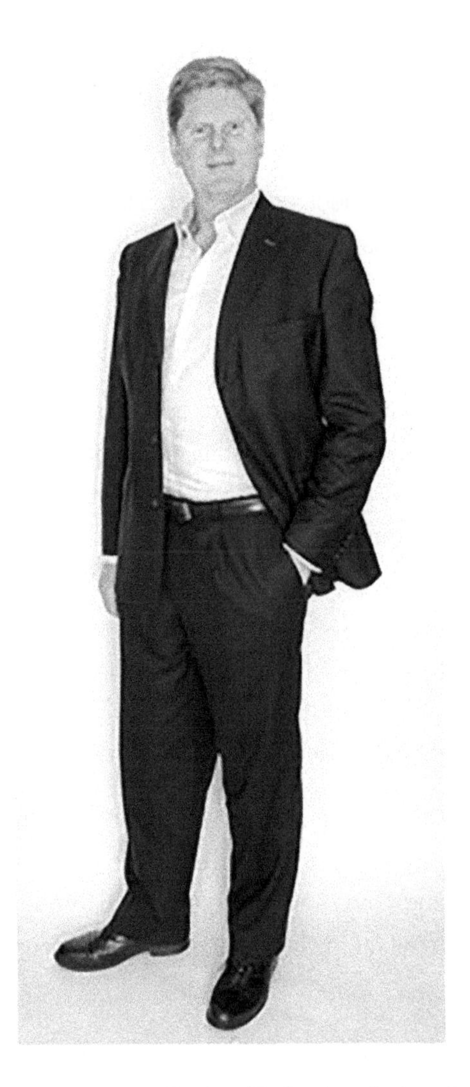

Matt looking 'normal' in Dress2Kill suit and iTailor shoes, both made-to-measure

Jeans

After two and a half years of buying oversized jeans via the internet, which, quite frankly, looked like something a clown would wear, my wife started researching again. Have you spotted a theme yet?

For Christmas 2014, my wife and parents bought me a voucher for Levi's Lot 1, a new made-to-measure service from Levi's. I actually cried at the thought of wearing jeans that actually fitted and disguised my lymphoedema. At my first appointment, I walked into the Regent Street, London store, a little uneasy amongst all these young, trendy assistants in their slim fit jeans. I felt immediately out of place and incredibly self-conscious, which was the polar opposite of what I was like before lymphoedema.

We were introduced to the Master Tailor, Elizabeth Radcliffe, and I explained my recent history with lymphoedema. She was so understanding, discreet and very keen to help me. Elizabeth, Lizzie as she prefers, took on board my objective to have a pair of jeans that looked as normal as possible, with both legs similar in size, so as not to draw attention to my F'leg. She quickly realised, on this occasion anyway, that I wasn't interested in the colour of the thread, or the style of button. I just wanted her to make me a pair of jeans that would hide the difference in leg size and help me to feel like 'me' again. Lizzie was certainly up for the challenge and was determined to produce a solution.

A few weeks later, the beautifully packaged jeans arrived at my home from Levi's and I was so excited to try them on. Lizzie had achieved all my objectives. The jeans were fantastic, and I couldn't wait to see her again to order my next pair. That time, I did pay more attention to the detailing and made them even more personalised. I could be trendy too, even at my age, right?

By my next appointment with Lizzie, I was back to my old self and felt incredible. What lymphoedema?

It is with heartfelt gratitude, that I introduce the wonderful Elizabeth (Lizzie) Radcliffe, Master Tailor of Levi's Lot 1 London to tell us more about this life-enhancing made-to-measure service.

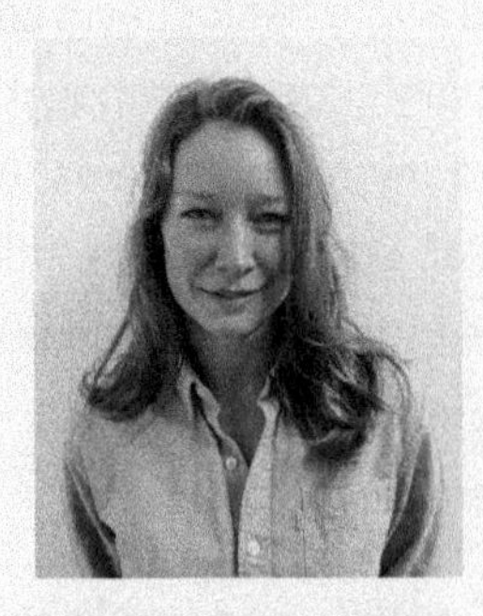

Elizabeth Radcliffe
Master Tailor
Levi's Lot 1

I still remember vividly when Matt walked into Lot 1, based then in the basement of the Levis' Regent Street store. For a man over 6ft tall, he walked with hunched shoulders, head cowed and seemed to lack the confidence you might usually see in a man of that stature. His appointment had actually been bought as a gift from his wife who knew how much he had struggled with getting jeans to fit from a shop floor.

We spoke at length about the requirements for his jeans - both in terms of look and dimensions but I was left with a feeling that the best thing these jeans could do for him was to make him look like everyone else - a rarity in the bespoke clothing world! Fairly often we are asked to make garments that stand out or are decidely different to those that you can buy off the shelf. It made me even more aware of how democratic jeans as a garment are. To this end, we used a Levis classic denim, with a colourway to match how the jeans would be produced in a factory.

Matt mentioned having had jeans or trousers made before, but that the tailors tried to 'fit' each leg resulting in a garment that actually drew attention to the lymphoedema rather than distracting from it.

The denim we use at Lot 1 is heavier than average meaning these jeans hold their shape well and hang rather than cling. We decided to make only minor differences between the left and right leg so the overall appearance was of two legs that looked the same.

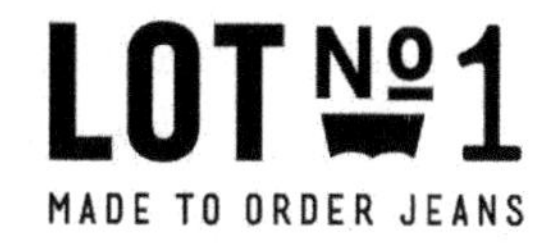

The process at Lot 1 requires you to have a fitting after the intial consultation (where you choose all the jeans details - denim/ threads colours/ button and rivet choices/ leather patch/ fit style etc) where you can try on the jeans you have chosen in your personal fit. Here we fine tune the fit and a few weeks later we would have the jeans ready for collection or to be posted out. If I recall correctly we posted these out to Matt so at that time I didn't get to see them on him. A few days after we shipped them we had a phone call from Vicki to inform us that the jeans fitted well and Matt was happy. It didn't hit home to me though, how important this was until a month or so later Matt happened to be in London and popped in to see us.

I didn't recongise the man that walked over. He walked with confidence, dare I say swagger (!) head held high and you would never have guessed that underneath those jeans he was hiding lymphoedema. We have made a few jeans for customers with medical problems - colostomy bags, amputees and other lymphoedema sufferers as a result of Matt's publicity for Lot 1, but it is Matt that sticks in my mind as the most memorable. To see that change in person's self esteem through a garment I made is an incredibly emotional feeling and still brings a tear to my eye to this day (6 years ago). I guess it is something that until that point I took for granted, being able to walk into a shop and pretty much fit into any garment there.

Through a feature that Matt and I collaborated on, both for the Lymphline blog and the Levis' website we have received commisions from a few more clients with the same condition. Not everyone tells us outright of their condition, it is a personal thing after all, but we know that we are enriching their lives through the work we do. What an intensely rewarding feeling that is.

We have a variety of selvedge denims to chose from and have added a few with a low stretch content in response to clients requests. We carry predominantly blue denims, a few blacks, some white shades and even a green and a red so there is something to suit most people's tastes. We can now offer a stonewashing service also.

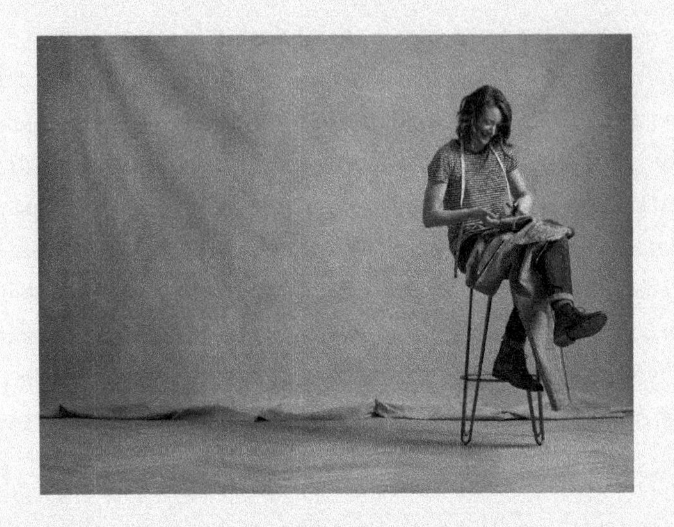

Elizabeth Radcliffe - Master Tailor, Levi's Lot 1

There are twenty thread colours to choose from and you can have up to five different colours throughout the jean. We have recently added 13 more 'red' tab colours including a rainbow tab to celebrate Pride, in addition to the classic red, black, white or navy traditional colours for tabs. We make you a paper pattern which we keep on file, allowing you to order again based off the same fit. All the jeans are personalised and editioned meaning you are truly getting a unique garment.

Alterations and repairs are included as part of the service, and we always love to see an old jean come back in and tell it's story through the wear lines. There are five of us in the team currently so each garment feels like an old friend.

They are an investment but given the denim we use and the attention to detail myself and the other Lot 1 tailors give to each pair I truly believe they merit the cost. Before I spoke to Vicki and met Matt, I had never heard of lymphoedema and I am delighted to be able to help people with this disease by creating perfectly fitted bespoke jeans. Jeans that you will have and cherish for life.

Thank you for taking the time to write this Lizzie, just at the incredibly busy time when the store reopened after the Covid-19 lockdown ended in May 2021.

For more information, visit their website *www.levi.com* or email *mastertailorlondon@levi.com*.

To raise awareness of lymphoedema, in August 2015, I wrote a blog for the Levi's website which reached a global audience and it is still on the site today, if you wish to read it. Apologies for the long link: *https://www.levistrauss.com/2015/08/24/at-last-the-perfect-pants/*.

To inform other people with lymphoedema of the Levi's Lot 1 service, I wrote an article for the LSN Winter 2015 Lymphline newsletter. Hopefully, that successfully covered both markets.

Lizzie really is a wonderful lady who is so kind and supportive, both at the time of our first meeting and ever since. We are currently in talks to provide an attractive discount to those signed up as free members to my website *www.lymphoedemaunited.com*.

In the past, I have tended to look at the cost and shy away from spending a lot of money on me. There always seems to be more important things to spend that amount of money on. Wrong! Start with you. Put yourself and your mental wellbeing first. Remember the saying when flying in an airplane, "in the event of an emergency, pull down and apply your own oxygen mask first before helping others". That justifies a top tip in my opinion.

Top Tip #35: Put yourself first. Remember "in the event of an emergency, pull down and apply your own oxygen mask first before helping others".

If you are still not convinced, apply the maths and divide the cost by the number of times you are likely to wear the garment. This will give you the 'cost per wear' and that figure should help you with your decision.

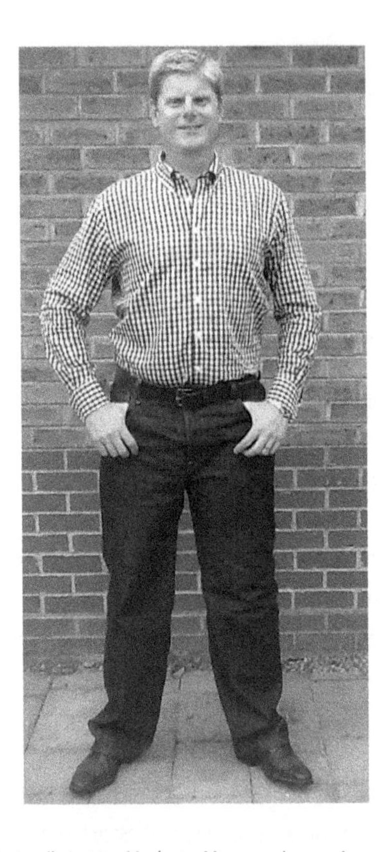

Matt in Levi's Lot 1 – Made-to-Measure Jeans: August 2015

Shirts & Jackets

I am almost certain that it's as difficult for a person with upper limb lymphoedema to find shirts, blouses and jackets, as it is for a person with lower limb lymphoedema to source trousers and jeans.

Although I have never purchased made-to-measure shirts online, I was pleased to see that iTailor provides bespoke custom-made shirts and blouses from £29.99 upwards. There is a comprehensive range available for men *www.itailor.com* and for women *www.itailor.com/collection/women/*.

iTailor also produce made-to-measure suits, but I haven't experienced this service, so I can't say for sure how good it is. However, if the shoes are anything to go by, this is worth exploring further.

I am sure there will be other websites, local tailors and seamstresses, who will be able to create a style of custom-fit clothes that you are happy with and that make you feel, well, like *you* again.

Socks

With lower limb lymphoedema, I found that my usual socks were too tight and would leave an indentation on my leg, with the elastic causing a kind of tourniquet effect. This is not good for my lymphatic drainage. Lymph fluid must travel up my leg, which already has its challenges, and I doubt I was helping my lymphatic system by strangulating it with tight-topped socks.

The internet is a wonderful thing when you know where to look. Could it be as easy as searching 'soft top socks'? Well, yes, it is as simple as that. There are various online shops selling such garments for men and women. Examples are: *www.softtopsocks.co.uk*, *www.hj.co.uk/softtop* , *www.sockshop.co.uk/* and *www.socksnob.co.uk/* or we can support the High Street by visiting shops like Marks & Spencer, or similar.

I was recently bought the stereotypical Christmas stocking filler present from my parents. Yes, you guessed it, socks. But not just any ordinary socks, my parents don't do ordinary. This was a three-pack of bamboo socks, which SockShop stock (great tongue twister!). Yes, you read this correctly, these are socks made from bamboo! I can vouch for the description that SockShop put on their website *www.sockshop.co.uk*, that "*as well as being incredibly soft, bamboo has many natural qualities that lend themselves perfectly to socks. Bamboo is two to three degrees cooler in warm weather and also very warm in cold weather, because its fibre micro-structure is filled with various micro-gaps and micro-holes. Bamboo is also three to four times more absorbent than cotton, and wicks away moisture from the skin, keeping feet fresh and dry*". Now that all sounds just the ticket for me with lower limb lymphoedema and I have to say, they are extremely comfortable, especially when I wear my comfy Skechers. What's happening to me!!!

Another online company specialising in a wide range of bamboo clothing, including socks, is BAM *www.bambooclothing.co.uk*.

The Overall Result = Much improved Self Confidence & Higher Self-esteem

I am now fortunate enough to have several pairs of Lot 1 jeans, a couple of suits and trousers, a selection of smart and comfy shoes, plus many pairs of soft top socks, of course. I have to say that wearing clothes that fit properly again has absolutely transformed me, mentally as well as physically. I am back to my old confident self and whilst I still have lymphoedema in my left leg, it doesn't notice as much as it did before. I am 100% certain that wearing made-to-measure clothes and shoes as well as my made-to-measure stockings, has increased my self-esteem immeasurably. This has made such a positive difference to my life, to the point that prior to all these positive changes, I wouldn't have been able to speak about lymphoedema to a small group of people, let alone feature in the Daily Mail, write a blog, write a newsletter article, appear in Professor Mortimer's book, be interviewed on the radio, oh and write this book and produce a website!

Top Tip #36: To justify the cost of buying bespoke clothes or shoes, calculate the cost divided by the number of times you will wear it = 'cost per wear.' Then apply increased self-esteem, greater confidence, feeling great, looking good...shall I go on?

Lymphoedema United - Members discounts

As you may have gathered by now, my other project is creating a new free membership website called *www.lymphoedemaunited.com*. The site is a platform to unite people living with lymphoedema, with medical experts, organisations and suppliers of specialist products for people with the condition. I will also include a section on lifestyle products, including clothes and shoes, plus anything else I find that may help us all to live better with lymphoedema.

I am in talks with all the companies mentioned in my book and more besides, to provide a unique discount code to members of Lymphoedema United. Keep an eye on the website, or even better, sign up as a free member today and opt in to receive emails and I will keep you posted of all the exciting developments. You can also follow us via social media platforms: Facebook, Twitter, Instagram, LinkedIn and YouTube.

Top Tip #37: Invest in yourself and improve your mental wellbeing by purchasing perfectly fitting made-to-measure clothes and shoes.

17

PUMP DOWN THE VOLUME

"The pump fills the air chambers in a sequence that stimulates drainage of lymphatic fluid."

—Naomi Northen-Ellis,
Director of Compression Therapy UK Ltd

Sorry, I couldn't resist the play on words with the title. It took me back to 1988 and strutting my stuff on the dance floors to the MARRS song "Pump up the volume, when the song beat goes like this...." Except, in this case, the purpose of the compression pump is to reduce the volume, but if I have to explain the joke, then I guess it wasn't funny to begin with.

There are many versions of compression pumps available on the market and although costly, they may be a wise investment in the self-management of lymphoedema. Naomi Northen-Ellis will explain more about compression pumps shortly and will do a far better job of that than I, so I won't steal her thunder. What I can do, is provide first-hand experience of using several pumps over the years from various manufacturers and explain how effective they were for me.

The first time I used a compression pump, was as part of Decongestive Lymphatic Therapy (DLT). On removal of the Multi-Layer Lymphoedema Bandaging (MLLB), my therapist would use a compression pump to simulate Manual Lymphatic Drainage (MLD) for a 45-minute period, three times per week, during the three-week treatment period. This allowed her time to write up the paperwork, catch up on emails and have a well-deserved cuppa, while I was relaxing in the comfortable recliner chair listening to the gentle, rhythmical humming and puffing noises of the pump.

In my case, I wore the inflatable blue leg sleeve or trouser, just on my affected left leg, with around eight to 10 tubes connected to two plugs that went into the machine. It was quite a sight, and I am so glad there were one-way privacy windows in the treatment room, at least that's what they told me at the time.

The 45-minute programme starts with the machine pumping air into specific pockets of the leg trouser, inflating and deflating at the top of the leg first and then gradually moving the starting point further down the leg until it reaches the foot. Once at the foot, the air pockets inflate and deflate sequentially upwards along the lower leg, the knee and upper leg, putting a comfortable and noticeable amount of pressure on the leg, essentially massaging the lymph fluid from the ankle to the groin area. It is very pleasant and although you cannot see what's happening, you can feel, or at least imagine, that the pump is pushing the lymph to the highest drainage point. It was impossible to gauge how much the pump reduced the volume in my leg, as it was a contributory part of the DLT process. However, this combination always resulted in an impressive reduction in volume, often reducing the volume from almost 50% to 35% more than my good, right leg. The frustration was that my leg would soon rebound in size, even when wearing a stocking with the highest level of compression, class 4S. Perhaps this shouldn't have been a surprise in my case. Professor Mortimer, Dr Gordon and I had exhausted all conservative methods to reduce and, more importantly for me, successfully maintain the reduction in volume. My leg always tended to rebound soon after any treatment, which was why surgery was a last throw of the dice for me.

I next used a compression pump in 2018. On this occasion, my local therapist arranged for me to attend the clinic and use a Hivermat pump for 45-minutes for four consecutive Fridays in April.

Most recently in April 2021, after several conversations with Naomi Northen-Ellis about my projects, she offered me a two-week trial of the Lympha Press compression pump from her company, Compression Therapy UK Ltd. I explained my history with lymphoedema, including the unplanned surgical removal of my inguinal lymph nodes on the left side of my groin, Lymph Node Transfer and Liposuction surgery. After listening intently, Naomi proposed supplying me with multi-chamber trouser garments, instead of the single leg that I had used previously. Her rationale for this, was that the single trouser would only pump the fluid up to my groin area and if the lymph nodes had been removed, combined with the sclerosis in the surrounding tissue, where would the fluid go? The trouser garment came up above the groin to the abdomen, which means that the fluid should bypass the groin and head towards the abdomen to assist drainage. That sounded like a very logical plan to me, and I willingly accepted the two-week trial.

The machine was delivered to my home by Royal Mail with instructions over the phone from Naomi on how to set the correct pressure. Having done this before, I was looking for a before and after comparison to see how effective this pump with trousers was for me. Using my lymphoedema measuring tape from Medi UK, I took some circumference measurements at my ankle, calf, knee and mid-thigh before starting the daily regime. Interestingly, I did see a reduction in the measurements by the end of the two-weeks. I can certainly see how a compression pump could be beneficial for people with lymphoedema, as part of a self-management regime at home, or as part of DLT.

Although I haven't ordered one yet, I may well invest in my own machine for the many years of lymphoedema I have ahead of me. Maybe one of the manufacturers will offer 0% finance for 48 months, like DFS does with their sofas, making it more affordable for the majority of us. I'll add that to my list when I next talk to Naomi and other pump suppliers.

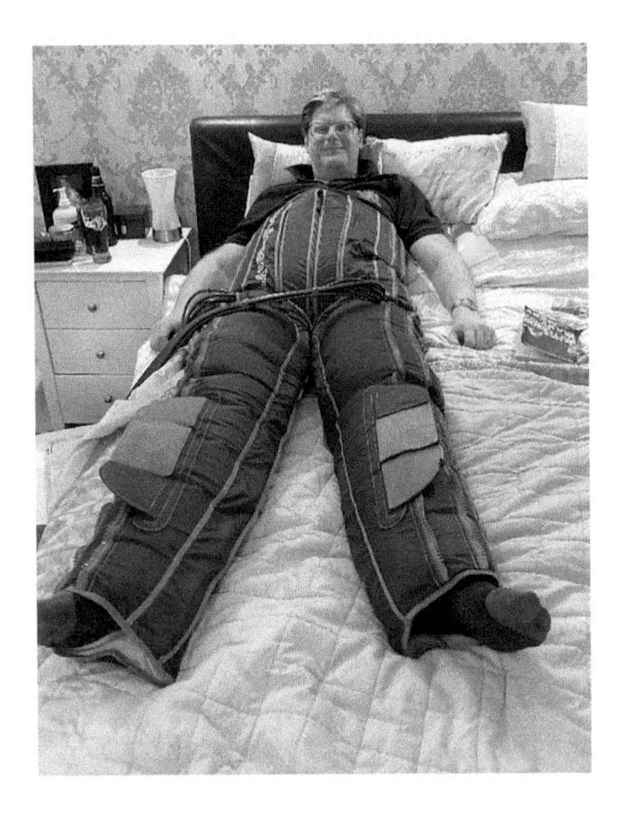

Matt trialling the Lympha Press Pump from Compression Therapy UK Ltd

(Note to self, remove the glass of lager when taking a photo in future – it was a hot day!)

I would like to thank Naomi for not just arranging a loan of her pump, but also for listening to my back-story and recommending the appropriate trouser garment. Her aim was to help *me* to live *better* with lymphoedema.

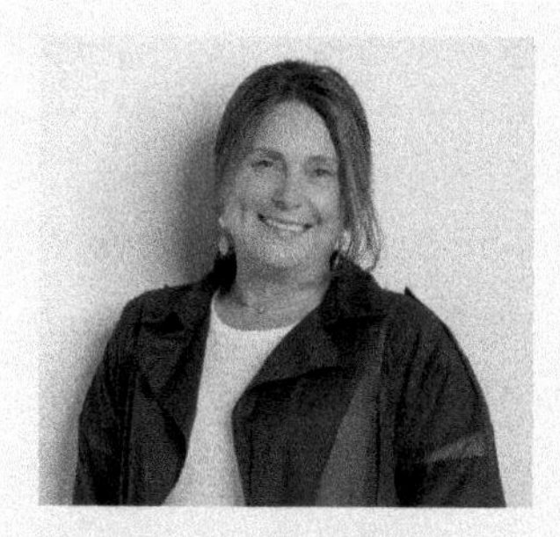

Naomi Northen-Ellis
Director/Owner, Compression Therapy UK Ltd

I have known of Matt's work within the lymphoedema community for a number of years. His willingness to share the story of his own lymphoedema, including his experiences with lymph node transfer and liposuction surgery, with others is admirable and I immediately loved his idea to write this book, particularly because it is written specifically for the patient, for the individual living with, and so often struggling with, the condition that is lymphoedema, on a day-to-day basis. I am confident that this book will give you an introduction to the many treatments and protocols that you may have heard mentioned, but not known where to access more facts, data and statistics.

For over 10 years I have been using a pump and I love it. It has given me the ability to take control in managing my own lymphoedema and I am passionate about encouraging others to do the same. It is so satisfying to witness how quickly they discover that regular use of a compression pump and garment, really does help. It not only improves their condition physically, but mentally too. It is such a liberating and cathartic experience for them, as they discover that they are in control of their own situation, it is no longer in control of them!

Intermittent Pneumatic Compression is an external pressure using compressed air and a pump. The compression pump works by alternately filling and deflating air chambers in a garment that is worn over the swollen area.

The pump fills the air chambers in a sequence that stimulates drainage of lymphatic fluid.

The rhythmic inflation and deflation of the chambers in the garments mimics the muscle pump action and promotes a strong venous return and lymphatic flow. It accelerates the removal of excess fluid in the interstitial tissues via the lymphatic system, reducing oedema volume. The intermittent compression helps soften fibrotic tissue, improves skin tone and assists lymph drainage that may have been compromised by fibrosis. The gentle pulsing action promotes relaxation whilst increasing lymphatic function during and post-treatment.

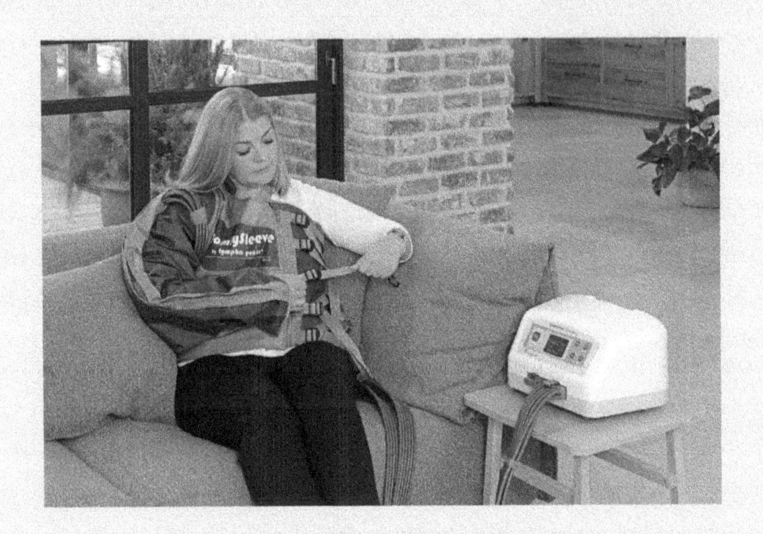

Lympha Press Pump for upper limb lymphoedema

The pressure in a pump is measured in 'milliliters of mercury' (mmHg) and pressures on most pumps can be selected between 20 – 90 mmHg. This range of pressure is appropriate for treatment of lymphoedema. Pressures should be chosen according to the patient's condition to encourage a healthy flow of lymph fluid.

We are not all created equal, and some people achieve better results with a slightly higher pressures and others with a lower pressure. For example, if the limb is hard and fibrotic a higher pressure will be required to soften the fibrotic tissue. Once that has been achieved the lymph will flow more freely and then pressures may be reduced. If a person is larger and has more fatty deposits in the tissue of the limb/s then a higher pressure may be required to stimulate the pump-like action and encourage the lymphatic flow and uptake of excess fluid from the interstitial tissues. Pressures should be re-evaluated when there is weight gain or loss and adjusted accordingly. It should be emphasized that the entire treatment should feel very relaxing and if there is any discomfort at all, that is an indication that the pressure may be too high and needs to be reduced.

Regular use of a pump brings many benefits:

- *Softening hard fibrotic areas*
- *Reducing swelling in the arms, legs and torso*
- *The repetitive massage action promotes a strong venous return and helps to achieve and maintain excellent skin health, thereby reducing the possibility of cellulitis infection*
- *Increasing mobility*
- *Decreasing feelings of heaviness or tightness*
- *Increasing the ability to move an affected arm or leg*
- *Increasing balance and ability to walk*
- *Decreasing pain*

If you have an MLD therapist that you are in regular contact with, then a good place to start would be to ask for their advice and guidance in approaching different suppliers.

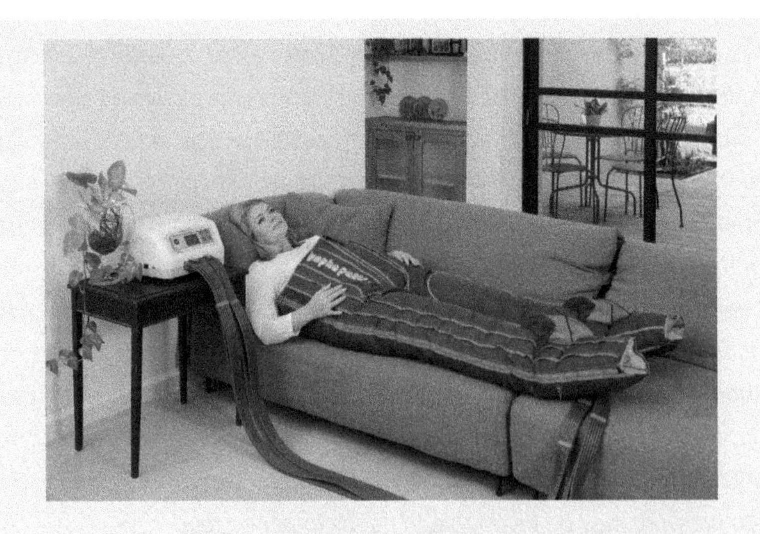

Lympha Press Pump for lower limb lymphoedema

Always make sure that you get a free trial before committing to a purchase and do not be pressured into making a purchase after a trial if you did not enjoy using it or found no benefit. You should expect to invest a considerable sum and it is wise to purchase the best you can afford. Use the web for research but buying something on-line just because it is cheap and looks the same as a more expensive product, does not mean that it is the same. Look upon the purchase as an investment into your long-term health and wellness; you will be using it daily and the product you choose should last you for years to come.

Select a product that you feel comfortable operating and that meets your needs in terms of your lymphoedema. Here are features to look for:

- *Multiple chambers: Avoid single chamber pumps that inflate the entire garment at once as they may cause wrong-way flow, like squeezing a tube of toothpaste in the middle. Multiple chambers enable a sequence from the hand or foot to the torso and assist in moving fluid to the lymphatic collection points in the torso.*

- *Overlapping chambers: The compression with overlapping chambers prevents gaps in treatment. Overlapping chambers follow multi-layer bandaging principles. Using garments that do not have overlapping chambers risks some areas going untreated.*
- *Treating the Torso: If you have lymphoedema in your torso, your upper arms or legs, you will need a full trouser or jacket garment to make sure fluid is moved beyond the affected area to the lymph nodes.*
- *The pump should fit your lifestyle. Make sure it is user friendly for your situation.*

Manage your expectations. Regular massage with a pump is extremely beneficial on many levels, the first priority is to keep the limb/s as healthy as possible. Softening fibrotic tissue and reducing volume can take time to achieve (although some people do get remarkable results very quickly).

Using a pump is not a substitute for wearing compression garments, although many people find they need a lighter compression when they use their pump regularly.

Keeping in touch with your care provider, be it through a private therapist or your local lymphoedema clinic or GP, will continue to be important to monitor and adjust your home program. If we all work together, we can and will, make a difference.

Thank you, Naomi, for supporting this project and helping lymphoedema sufferers. To find out more, visit *www.compressiontherapyuk.com*

Top Tip #38: Investigate whether a Compression Pump works for you, by arranging a two-week trial free of charge.

18

LYMPH NODE TRANSFER (LNT)

"LNT is usually reserved for those patients whose lymphoedema has progressed beyond the stage where LVA is possible."

—Professor Dominic Furniss DM MA MBBCh FRCS (Plast),
Professor of Plastic and Reconstructive Surgery

After a consultation meeting with Professor Mortimer on 26 October 2012, he wrote in his follow-up letter a clear explanation as to what I was dealing with. *"This type of lymphoedema requires high compression to stand any chance of reducing the size of the limb. I think compression garments, pneumatic compression pumps and wraps are going to be insufficient to make forward progress."*

This really limited my options somewhat to Multi-Layer Lymphoedema Bandaging (MLLB), which had shown excellent results in reduction initially, but which sadly were always short-lived as my leg would quickly rebound in the weeks following treatment. This wasn't really practical as a long-term solution and it was in March 2014, just over three years after my first appointment with Professor Mortimer, that he proposed surgery as the next step. He wrote to Mat Griffiths, a Consultant Plastic Surgeon at Broomfield Hospital in Chelmsford, Essex, asking him to see me *"for consideration of either LVA or perhaps Lymph Node Transfer given the fact that the fault appears to be at the level of the left ilioinguinal nodes."* LVA stands for Lymphovenous Anastomosis surgery as you probably know.

The response was surprisingly quick and I was invited to Broomfield Hospital for a CT and PDE (Photodynamic Eye) Scan in May 2014. Shortly afterwards in June 2014, I received a follow-up letter from Mat Griffiths. This was all moving unbelievably swiftly and my expectations were increasing due to the positive tone of his letter. He wrote:

"I have been reviewing your CT scan with my Radiologist Dr Railton and looking again at the investigations we have done with the photodynamic eye machine. You did have an impressive amount of scarring in the left groin in the subcutaneous tissues and as there is clearly a very focal element to your problem. I do think we should perhaps focus more on dealing with the scar area in the groin.

Reviewing your PDE scan, I think that with the kind of pattern you have in the ankle and leg, that finding useful lymphatics is going to be unlikely. Whereas if we release the scar in the groin and import functioning lymph nodes from the neck on the right side, I think this will be a better way to improve your lymphoedema. The scarring is obviously a result of the fact that it took seven weeks for your groin wound to heal.

As such, I recommend that we consider the scar in the left groin and then I will work in conjunction with a colleague of mine, Mr El-Muttardi, who is a Head and Neck Surgeon, who harvests the nodes for me in the neck area and then we can transplant these to the left groin once I have released the extensive scarring. As you have not had a lymph node clearance, as I tend to usually find in cancer patients, you have a lot more options in the groin with regards to vessels I can use to hook up the transplanted tissue which will make things slightly easier for both of us. The surgery will take around 4-5 hours and you will be in hospital for around 5 days. I took the liberty of speaking to my colleague about doing a joint case on a Friday when we are in adjacent theatres, so there will be some slightly logistical details to get around but when I have got some provisional dates from Mr El-Muttardi, then we will contact you to see if they are appropriate for your work."

Professor Mortimer had already advised me that after LNT surgery had been completed, liposuction would be an effective surgery to remove the remaining fat from my leg, caused by the lymphoedema. All was good and we had a plan of action. I had hope.

A few months before surgery, my leg measurements and volume were taken by one of the therapists at Broomfield Hospital, showing a 39% increase versus the right leg. This was the best size my left leg had been for quite some time now. Surgery was booked for August 2014 and I couldn't wait. I will share the outcome with you later!

I remember hearing from another surgeon that Broomfield Hospital no longer provides this service, which may explain why I didn't hear back from Mat Griffiths when I asked him to feature in this chapter. Instead, I contacted another expert in this field, Professor Dominic Furniss, Surgeon at the Oxford Lymphoedema Practice (OLP).

Professor Furniss' area of specialism is surgery for lymphoedema, including LVA, LNT and Liposuction. It is no surprise, therefore, that he was delighted to explain more about all three surgeries in the next few chapters, mainly to ensure that accurate information was made available to people with lymphoedema, who may be considering surgery.

I first met Professor Furniss several years ago when he made an interesting and informative presentation about these surgeries at an LSN Patient Conference. May I take this opportunity to thank him for the time he afforded me with both projects.

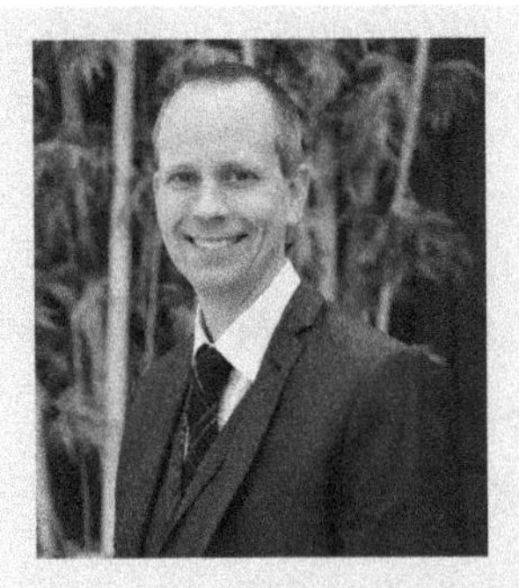

Professor Dominic Furniss DM MA MBBCh FRCS(Plast),
Professor of Plastic and Reconstructive Surgery
Oxford Lymphoedema Practice

Supermicrosurgical Lymphatic Reconstruction using Lymphaticovenous Anastomosis (LVA) or Lymph Node Transfer (LNT)

I was delighted when Matt asked me to contribute to this book, and his forthcoming website. I truly believe that only by informing the patient of all options available to them can they make a fully informed decision about their care. Too often, patients have come to me asking why their doctor or practitioner didn't inform them of our surgical service years ago, leaving them to suffer in isolation. It is only through initiatives like this that patients can be empowered.

Background

Before considering the role of supermicrosurgery in reconstruction of the lymphatic system, it is important to be clear on where the fluid in lymphoedema actually comes from. In a normal person, fluid is lost from the circulation as it passes through the capillaries of an arm or leg. This fluid is taken back by the lymphatic system to the blood system using a connection to the veins deep inside the neck.

Lymphoedema is a condition where an excess of fluid builds up in the arm or leg, usually because of impairment to the outflow of lymphatic fluid from the affected area. This causes excessive swelling, restricted movement, pain, recurrent episodes of severe infection (cellulitis), and subsequently a greatly decreased quality of life for the patient.

Lymphoedema may be primary or secondary, based on underlying cause. Primary lymphedema is caused by abnormal development of the lymphatic system. It can be present at birth, or develop later in life. In general, the failure of the lymphatics can either be in the microscopic capillaries, the lymph channels themselves, or in the lymph glands (so called lymph node sclerosis).

Most commonly in the western world, lymphoedema develops secondary to damage to normal lymphatics, from surgery (axillary or groin lymph node dissection), or radiotherapy. There is scarring of the lymphatic system in either the groin or armpit, which causes a blockage to the flow of lymph fluid back to the veins in the neck.

LNT Surgery

Lymph node transfer is a surgical technique where a "flap" or block of tissue which contains a number of lymph nodes is removed from elsewhere on the body and transplanted into the area that has lymphoedema. The blood vessels supplying the LNT are re-connected to a new blood supply using microsurgery. The areas that a transplant is often taken from are the neck area or inside the tummy (known as an omental flap). The omental flap is the slightly more complex of the two, and the surgeons performing this operation should be fully trained. Some surgeons take lymph nodes from the armpit or the groin, but this risks the patient developing lymphoedema in the arm or leg, respectively.

LNT is much more invasive than LVA. It requires a general anaesthetic, and usually a two-night hospital stay. There are greater risks in doing the surgery, including risks of general anaesthetic like getting a chest infection, or having a heart attack or stroke. Because of this increased risk, LNT is usually reserved for those patients whose lymphoedema has progressed beyond the stage where LVA is possible.

It is not fully understood how LNT works. Some theories include the release of growth factors that help stimulate lymphatic function and allow the lymph nodes to link up with the lymphatics in the surrounding tissue. Others believe there are naturally occurring microscopic LVAs within the lymph nodes themselves. However, it is evident that LNT can be helpful for those with lymphoedema, and some remaining lymphatic function. The effect of LNT on lymphoedema is usually not seen until several months after surgery, when the post-operative swelling starts to go down.

Thank you, Professor Furniss for your explanation of Lymph Node Transfer surgery. For more information, please visit Oxford Lymphoedema Practice website *www.olp.surgery* or contact Professor Furniss at *dominic@olp.surgery*.

As mentioned earlier, when my leg was measured at Broomfield Hospital in April 2014, my volume was looking good at 39% bigger than the right leg. Wow! If this surgery was a success, then we were aiming for between 20-25% as a target figure. Yes, I could definitely live with that, no problem at all.

I was told that the operation went as planned. Then, it was just a matter of time for the new lymph nodes from my neck to bed-in to my groin area, connect to the lymphatics and start draining, simply speaking, of course. Post-surgery measurements were taken and as expected, due to the post-op swelling in my leg, the volume had increased to 40%. I was told that a reduction in volume may take around four to six weeks after surgery. This all seemed totally plausible to me due to the intensive and intrusive nature of the procedure. My groin area was a little sore but more noticeable was the heavy numbness in my neck and shoulder. This was due to the nerves being cut in the process of accessing my lymph nodes. It took many weeks for the numbness to ease, although not completely. My recollection is that I still had slight tingling in this area for almost a year after surgery. It didn't bother me, but the nerve damage was a constant reminder of the surgery.

In September 2014 almost a month post-surgery, I was invited back to Broomfield Hospital for a check-up and to be remeasured for the before and after size comparison. It was evident before the nurse even got her tape measure out of her pocket, that my leg looked so much better than before. Knowing this in advance, I was so ecstatic that I took Mat Griffiths a very nice bottle of red wine as a gift to say thank you. I also sponsored him for a charity bike ride he was doing. I think I had developed a bit of a man-crush to be honest. I wasn't quite expecting the result that followed though, an amazing reduction in volume to 32%. I had only ever experienced this once or twice as a result of Decongestive Lymphatic Therapy (DLT) and Multi-Layer Lymphoedema Bandaging (MLLB). However, I believed that this would remain at this size. I wanted to hug everyone, in fact, I probably did!

However, I still feel immense sadness and disappointment as I write this because, by the time of my next appointment in November 2014, my leg had rebounded, significantly. No matter what steps I had taken to control it: wearing Class 4S flat knit stocking; Class 2 toe cap; Eto shorts; applying compression wraps in the evening; and performing Self-Lymphatic-Drainage, I couldn't stop the rebound.

It was no surprise to me that the new measurements would show an increase in volume, I just wasn't prepared for by just how much, 47%. My leg had returned to its typical size before starting DLT and MLLB treatment. Any reassurance that Mat and the nurse gave me fell on deaf ears. I cannot adequately describe to you how deflated I was as I walked back to the car park. I remember sitting in my car, feeling numb and emotional. I had a good cry before setting off on the 90-minute drive back home. The follow-up letter from Mat Griffiths tried to give me hope by saying and I quote *"As discussed, we do still have the option of attempting a lymphovenous anastomosis and especially in the calf/knee area where things are softer. I think this would stand a better chance of providing some benefit."* LVA surgery would only be a consideration once an MRI scan of the deep lymphatics was done, enabling Mat to assess whether the LVA surgery would be worthwhile or not. This scan was never forthcoming.

Time passed by and after correspondence between Professor Mortimer, Glen Brice, (Clinical Nurse Specialist in Genetics at the St George's Hospital) and Mat Griffiths, Mat responded in his letter dated August 2015 *"I think LVAs are unlikely to have made any benefit, but it would be good to explore all avenues."* It was also explained in his letter that Broomfield Hospital didn't have the funding for the machine that could perform the MRI scan to assess my deep lymphatics. It was clear to me, that this would take some years to proceed, if at all, and if it did proceed the expectation of success was low. The last time I visited Broomfield Hospital was in February 2015, for a check-up and remeasuring. The volume had increased to the highest level EVER at a distressing 58%. I had not only gone backwards, but my leg was the biggest it had ever been. It was at this point that my optimism and hope for any kind of solution began to dissolve rapidly. The shape and size of my leg were a constant reminder that even surgery had failed, and I couldn't see a way forward. What a rollercoaster of emotions.

By then I was really struggling to walk properly due to the extra weight of my left leg, which was putting tremendous pressure on my back, causing constant pain. I continued to exercise to strengthen my core and keep fit. It was during a game of golf with three other businessmen, that a bolt of pain struck me after teeing off on the 14th hole and I had to stop instantly. I couldn't even walk back to the clubhouse and had to call the pro shop for someone to come and collect me with a golf cart. How embarrassing and how debilitating. Was my beloved golf the next sacrifice I had to make?

My GP arranged for me to have an X-ray and MRI scan which showed that I had a disc bulge in the right side of my lower back. I was told that this was brought on by the way I was walking due to my heavy left leg, as the right side of my body was over-compensating for my left side. I was referred to a specialist physiotherapist who instantly spotted that my gait was out of line. I had many physio sessions, yet the pain wouldn't budge, so I was also referred to the Pain Clinic at the local hospital for a steroid injection. Significant lifestyle changes had to be made, including selling my dream car that I had worked so hard to buy, a beautiful black convertible. Golf was not on the radar for the foreseeable future, but much more importantly than that, I wasn't great company when spending time with family and friends, due to the pain. The ongoing treatment I was having was placing tremendous pressure on the relationship with my business partner. Things were very tough indeed and I was struggling to see how, or where, any improvement to my leg, back, or state of mind would come from.

19

LYMPHOVENOUS ANASTOMOSIS (LVA)

"LVA surgery has the big advantage of being very minimally invasive."

—PROFESSOR DOMINIC FURNISS DM MA MBBCH FRCS(PLAST),
PROFESSOR OF PLASTIC AND RECONSTRUCTIVE SURGERY

As you read in the previous chapter, Professor Mortimer referred me to Mat Griffiths – Consultant Plastic Surgeon at Broomfield Hospital in Chelmsford, Essex, to assess the viability for me to have Lymphovenous Anastomosis or Lymph Node Transfer surgery. Mat's recommendation was for me to have the latter, as he wrote in a follow up letter *"finding useful lymphatics is going to be unlikely"* making LVA less effective for my circumstances.

Therefore, LVA surgery wasn't suitable for me and it remains the only lymphoedema treatment or surgery that I am aware of, that I haven't experienced.

As LVA is a recognised surgery for people with lymphoedema, it would be remiss of me to exclude it from my book, just because I haven't had personal experience of it. LVA could be a suitable option for other people with lymphoedema.

To explain more about LVA, I am delighted to introduce you once again to an expert in this field, Professor Dominic Furniss.

Professor Furness is a Surgeon at the Oxford Lymphoedema Practive (OLP) and he was delighted to explain more about Lymphovenous Anastomosis surgery in this chapter, mainly to ensure that accurate information was made available to people with lymphoedema, who may be considering this surgery.

Warning: the image provided is not for the squeamish.

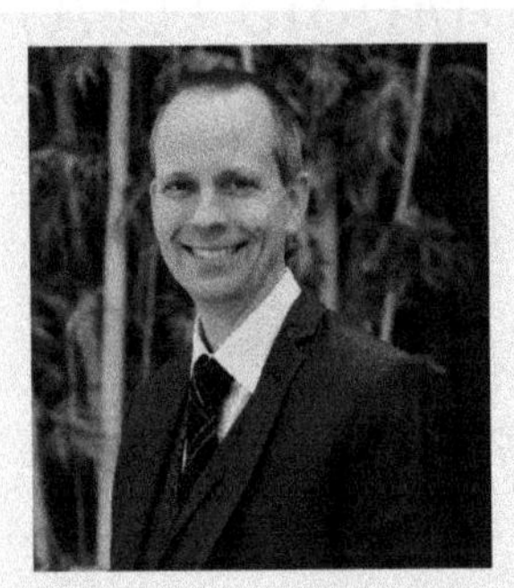

Prof Dominic Furniss DM MA MBBCh FRCS(Plast),
Professor of Plastic and Reconstructive Surgery
Oxford Lymphoedema Practice

LVA Surgery

The idea of LVA surgery is to connect functioning lymphatic channels within the arm or leg directly to small veins. This allows the lymphatic fluid to drain back into the veins directly, without having to get past the blockage higher up in the system. It is just like building a bypass to relieve pressure on a road that is too small for the amount of traffic it carries.

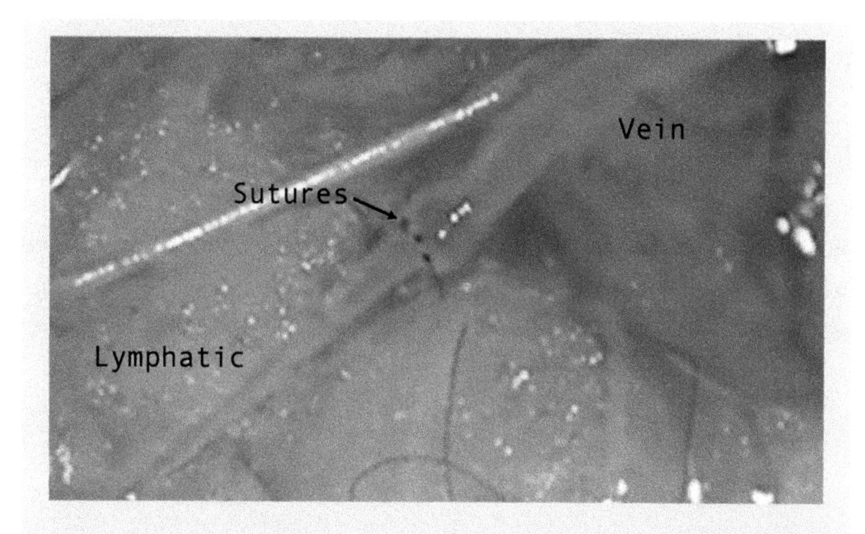

A lymphaticovenular anastomosis. The delicate lymphatic contains lymph fluid stained blue using a special dye. It has been sutured to the slightly larger vein, and the blue-stained lymphatic fluid can be seen passing into the vein, relieving the lymphoedema

LVA surgery has the big advantage of being very minimally invasive. It is usually carried out under local anaesthetic, and the patient can go home the same day. The incisions in the arm or leg are only around 2-4cm long, and heal well. The risk of complications is low.

However, LVA surgery is very technically demanding, and requires surgeons to be specially trained to a very high level. The lymphatic channels and veins that we use for LVA surgery are usually between 0.3 and 0.8 mm in diameter, and the thread used to stitch them together is invisible to the naked eye. We use powerful operating microscopes with special instruments to enable us to successfully perform the surgery.

LVA has been shown in multiple clinical studies to improve both the symptoms of lymphoedema, like swelling, pain, and restricted movement, and also to prevent worsening of lymphoedema in the longer term. It also improves quality of life in people with lymphoedema. Some patients are able to no longer wear their compression garments after surgery, and many can reduce the amount that they wear them. Importantly, LVA reduces the risk of developing cellulitis, a dangerous infection of the skin that is more likely in someone with lymphoedema.

For more information about LVA, please visit Oxford Lymphoedema Practice website *www.olp.surgery* or contact Professor Furniss at *dominic@olp.surgery*.

20

LIPOSUCTION IN LYMPHOEDEMA

> *"When undertaken by an experienced team, liposuction for lymphoedema gives highly predictable results that are long lasting, and greatly enhance quality of life for patients."*
>
> —Professor Dominic Furniss DM MA MBBCh FRCS(Plast),
> Professor of Plastic and Reconstructive Surgery

I would suggest getting a cup of tea or coffee for this one, as it's quite a long chapter with much to tell.

In Chapter 18, I explained my experience of Lymph Node Transfer surgery which, frustratingly, didn't have the desired results. The outcome meant that the size of my leg actually *increased* to the largest size EVER, with a volume of 58% in February 2015. The difference in size and weight of my left leg put tremendous pressure on my right leg, hip and lower back, which were overcompensating for my left side. When walking, I was almost swinging my left leg, and when stationary, I stood lop-sided to the right. It transpired that I had a disc bulge in my lower back on the right side, which explained the level of pain I was in. A steroid injection administered by the Pain Clinic did help for a while, but it just deferred the problem. I have to admit, these were tough times. The size of my leg and the back pain were all consuming and I couldn't see a solution to this problem. Cue Professor Mortimer.

At my next consultation with Professor Mortimer, my desperation was evident. I could see that he understood and genuinely empathised with the position I was now in. Previous scans had shown that due to my damaged lymphatics, LVA was unsuitable for me and unlikely to be successful. We both knew that this situation couldn't continue indefinitely without further intervention and that was when he suggested that we investigate the suitability of liposuction surgery.

He explained that the purpose of liposuction in my case, would be to reduce the volume of the lymphatic 'fat' in my left leg, thus reducing the weight, which in turn would help to rebalance my gait and ease the pressure on my back, reducing the aggravation on the disc bulge. The results of yet another lymph scan had shown that *"the main drainage routes do not appear to be functional, and drainage is through the multiple small collateral routes particularly in the skin. Function was insufficient for the dye to reach the lymph glands in the groin and so they were not imaged".*

Late November 2015, Professor Mortimer wrote a letter to request an appointment for me to see my Consultant, Dr Kristiana Gordon and Ms Catherine Milroy – Consultant in Plastic and Reconstructive Surgery at St George's Hospital, to investigate the suitability of liposuction. The meeting was soon set for March 2016. Liposuction was the only option left to improve my lymphoedema, my quality of life and my mental wellbeing, so I had nothing to lose.

Spring came, daffodils were in bloom and on 18th March 2016 I met with Dr Gordon and Ms Milroy for an in-depth conversation about liposuction/

suction-assisted lipectomy. After an examination, they deemed that my leg was suitable for the surgery, because my thigh was exclusively fatty with no pitting oedema. From the knee to mid-shin, I had severe pitting lymphoedema that then tapered off to reveal minimal/mild lymphoedema of the foot and ankle region.

Ms Milroy explained the process and the pros and cons of liposuction, including a warning that the pain was like being run over by a bus, twice! Oh well, no pain no gain as the saying goes. Another point they raised was that post-surgery there would be a need to wear compression garments 24/7 every day thereafter, to prevent the leg from refilling with lymph fluid which could turn into fatty, fibrous tissue once again.

It was made very clear to me, both at the meeting and in the follow-up letter, that liposuction was not a cure for lymphoedema, but it would reduce my massive leg volumes. This, in turn, would reduce my musculoskeletal problems, including hip pain and tilting pelvis, therefore improving my mobility and quality of life. We all agreed that this was the best solution for me, and a new plan was made. However, there were no guarantees that this would proceed. Dr Gordon and Ms Milroy had to make a strong case in their application to the Clinical Commissioning Group (CCG) to secure funding, allowing it to proceed on the NHS. Very tight NHS budgets meant that this was not a done deal by any means.

Before I was deemed suitable for liposuction surgery, a treatment plan had to be implemented and achieved, to reduce the amount of fluid in my leg and leave behind the fatty tissue. If this was successful, then it would improve the chances that I was eligible for liposuction surgery. Simultaneously, Dr Gordon and Ms Milroy were waiting to hear whether the funding had been obtained from the CCG or, indeed, declined. If the volume of fluid was not reduced to a satisfactory level, then the surgery would not proceed anyway, so the next six to nine months proved to be vital.

There were too many 'ifs' for my liking and the odds seemed stacked against me: If we could significantly reduce the fluid in my leg; if my leg was deemed suitable for liposuction; if funding was approved by the CCG; if I was able to ever get my life back to some degree of normality. If, if, if, if. That's a lot of ifs!

The plan to get me and my leg match-fit for liposuction surgery was as follows:

- Daily intensive Multi-Layer Lymphoedema Bandaging (MLLB) to reduce the volume
- Then, more aggressive combinations of garments, such as layering of thigh length and two layers below knee, adding a lower leg garment to maintain the reduced volume
- Wear compression garments 24/7. Class 4S during the day and Class 2 or 3 at night
- Lose weight, improve fitness, healthy diet, all to get my body in the best shape possible.

In October, I received a letter inviting me to an appointment with Dr Gordon and Ms Milroy at St George's on 18th November 2016. Thankfully, they informed me that the CCG had approved funding for the surgery and subject to how well my leg had responded to the intensive treatment, we were good to go!

Now for the examination. I went behind the curtain, took off my shoes, jeans, socks and stocking, got onto the couch and exclaimed "I'm ready"! So much depended on this examination and as Dr Gordon poked and prodded my leg in search of any pitting in my leg, you could have heard a pin drop.

Ms Milroy then assessed my leg and concluded that it was now suitable for surgery to be effective and, therefore, she would proceed with liposuction/ suction-assisted lipectomy, possibly as soon as January 2017, just under two months' time. I am getting chills whilst writing this, as I can remember being so very grateful to both of them for obtaining funding and agreeing to proceed with this potentially life-changing surgery.

Ms Milroy explained that she would initially operate on the lower leg, focusing on the calf and knee and, if time permitted, she would work on my thigh. If there wasn't time, however, then liposuction on the thigh would be deferred to a later date. Liposuction cannot be performed on the foot and ankle region, which was not an issue for me as this area had very minimal swelling. She warned me, again, that liposuction is very painful and that my leg was likely to swell significantly in the post-operative period. In addition, other possible risks included nerve damage and infection. It was made clear to me that by having liposuction, I was precluding myself from future treatment with LVA surgery as liposuction will damage any draining pathways. This was not a problem for me as we knew I was not suitable for LVA anyway.

My admission date was booked for 10th January 2017 for a 14-day stay at St George's Hospital. For the first seven days, I would have intensive bandaging daily, prior to surgery on 17th. I would then stay in hospital for a further seven days for pain control and further bandaging. Well, this was probably the best news I had received in years and it was the perfect early Christmas present. After the appointment, my wife and I had a celebratory lunch with a bottle of fizz and then, to help stay fighting fit for the surgery, I did not touch another drop of alcohol prior to my admission. OK, the only exceptions being a tipple on Christmas Day and then again on New Year's Eve.

I went into hospital at my lowest weight for years, 16½ stones. I looked and felt great. My spirits and expectations were soaring high and I was really looking forward to having surgery. I know that sounds an odd thing to say, but if you have read all the previous chapters, then I am sure that you will understand my excitement. This time, surgery would work, and I would be me again. Wouldn't I?

Before I continue with my liposuction experience and the recovery that followed, I would like to thank the fabulously talented Surgeon, Ms Catherine Milroy. Ms Milroy, like so many other medical professionals, is constantly busy and any spare time is incredibly rare and extremely precious. After inviting her to write in this chapter, she said that she would try her best, but was frantically busy with many other projects. Unfortunately, time ran out and I needed to publish the book without her much anticipated contribution. I will include it on my website should I receive it in future.

I am very grateful, again, to Professor Dominic Furniss, who stepped into the breach at short notice to explain the process involved with liposuction/ suction-assisted lipectomy, in addition to the benefits and risks associated with this type of surgery.

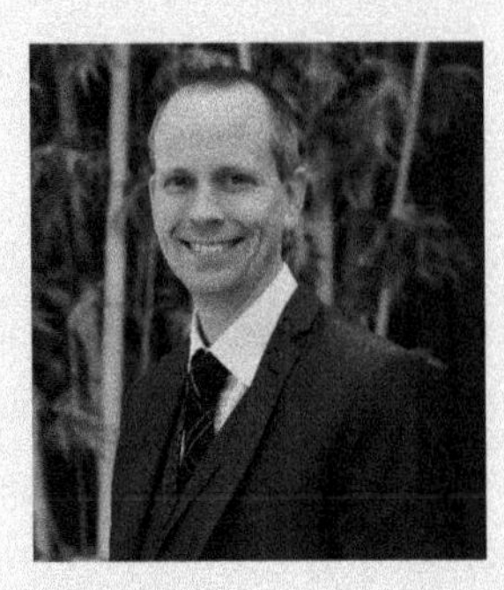

Professor Dominic Furniss DM MA MBBCh FRCS(Plast),
Professor of Plastic and Reconstructive Surgery
Oxford Lymphoedema Practice

Liposuction for lymphoedema

The fluid that accumulates in lymphoedema is not simply water. It contains a complex mix of proteins, growth factors, and pro-inflammatory factors. These factors cause the fat cells underneath the skin to get bigger, independent of a person putting on weight. They also cause fibrosis (scarring) of these subcutaneous tissues. Over time, the lymphoedema transforms from being mainly fluid (pitting), to mainly fat and scar tissue (non-pitting).

Reconstructive surgical options such as LVA and LNT are designed to improve fluid drainage from an area of lymphoedema. These options will be ineffective in reducing the size of a limb if the predominant cause of the swelling is fat. It is therefore imperative to determine the amount of fat and fluid in a limb before surgery, and this is achieved with a special MRI scan that can quantify both fat and fluid independently.

If the predominant cause of swelling is fat, then an appropriate solution is liposuction for lymphoedema. In this procedure, under general anaesthetic, multiple tiny incisions are made in the arm or leg through which the excess fat is removed by suction. Measurements are taken beforehand, and precise volumes of fat are removed to balance the size of the limb to the normal side as much as possible.

Because the lymphatics are not reconstructed in any way, and the surgery causes swelling, there is an increased reliance on compression therapy after surgery. Typically, patients need to wear strong compression for 23 hours per day for at least the first year after surgery. After this, many patients need to continue to wear round the clock compression, but a lucky few can reduce the length of time they wear their garments.

Liposuction for lymphoedema is not the same as cosmetic liposuction and should only be undertaken by specialist surgeons specifically trained in this technique. The key to success is working closely with equally highly trained lymphoedema practitioners, as the requirement for compression in the first year after surgery is intensive, with many regular adjustments needed in order to maintain the surgical result. However, when undertaken by an experienced team, liposuction for lymphoedema gives highly predictable results that are long lasting, and greatly enhance quality of life for patients.

Thank you, Professor Furniss, for the invaluable insight into liposuction for lymphoedema patients. I am sure that the many people that you have helped with this surgery are truly grateful for your expertise. For more information, please visit Oxford Lymphoedema Practice website *www.olp.surgery* or contact Professor Furniss at *dominic@olp.surgery*.

Let's head back to 10th January 2017, when I *walked* into the Amyand Ward on St James' Wing of St George's Hospital, London. I emphasise walked as that was barely what it was. Due to severe lower back and hip pain, I was wincing as I hobbled into the ward like an elderly man. I felt like I was in the right place as I passed open rooms, each with six beds, occupied mainly by very senior gentlemen. I introduced myself to the first nurse I saw, who turned around with a beautiful, warm smile and replied with a cheerful *"Good morning, I'm Hope!".* Wow! This was a welcomed omen, and that her name described the most salient emotion that I was feeling, *hope*. Hope that this surgery would help me return to my normal life again.

After unpacking my bag and getting organised for my two-week vacation in Tooting's finest, it was time for my first test. Two nurses, one with a clipboard, the other with a stopwatch, led me to the entrance of the ward at the beginning of a long corridor, which transpired to be the start line. My test was to walk the length of the corridor and then back again, while the stopwatch was tracking how quickly I could do this. Prior to having lymphoedema and a bad back, I could have run several lengths without the need of a defibrillator. On around my eighth embarrassing and painful lap of sluggish shuffling up and down the corridor, the nurses' long shifts had ended, and the sister was calling lights out for bedtime! I jest, but I'm sure you get the gist of my joke.

On the morning of day two, Decongestive Lymphatic Therapy (DLT) began and every day thereafter for two weeks, one of the specialist lymphoedema therapists would provide Multi-Layer Lymphoedema Bandaging (MLLB) and Manual Lymphatic Drainage (MLD).

By the end of day two, the bedrest was having a miraculous effect on my back and the constant pain had begun to ease. I was not on any pain-killers, I think the combination of rest, comfortable elevation and regular movement was having the desired effect. Perhaps, the fact that I was de-stressing as well may have contributed too. I was able to walk a little easier, so on that day I took the opportunity to go to the M&S shop at the main entrance of the hospital, in my MLLB bandages. It's probably a 10-minute walk if taking the lift, which I did on that occasion and *only* on that occasion. I bought some oranges and lemons, some squash, anything to improve the taste of the tap water. In addition, I bought some sugar-free mints, bananas, apples, some unsalted nuts and a few car magazines. Sorted!

I quickly got into a daily routine, which included: reading books; a bit of walking; watching a film on my portable DVD player; more walking; listening to the radio; checking in at the office; even more walking, all in-between having the regular observational checks from the nurses. It felt strange being in hospital and not being unwell or injured. I was fine (there it is again) and so took the opportunity to get to know the nurses and kind of fend for myself whilst I could. This included refilling my jug with water and doing the same for the bedridden patients. I got my own towels from the storeroom, made my own hot drinks, essentially anything that I could do for myself to save the nurses a job, I would.

The objective of having DLT was to reduce as much of the fluid in my leg as possible, leaving just the fatty tissue caused by lymphoedema, for liposuction to remove. Exercise and movement are an important part of DLT therapy which I was strongly encouraged to do. My only other instruction was to elevate my legs in bed to improve drainage. Sitting down would result in the fluid draining downwards thus defeating the object. Therefore, I decided on a plan and on day three, I set the alarm on my phone every hour from 9am to 8pm. On the hour every hour, I would get up and walk up and down the length of the corridor for five minutes, counting how many laps I could do within the time, using the stopwatch on my phone. By day four, I would also walk down eight flights of stairs and then back up again, before returning to the ward. I did get some strange looks whilst pacing repeatedly with such a bulky leg covered in bandages, but that didn't faze me. It was all to improve the chances of a successful surgery and the only person to benefit from that was me.

I did five minutes of walking, every hour, eight times every day for seven days pre-op and then after a couple of days of post-surgery rest, I would start back up again. The number of laps gradually increased as the back pain gradually reduced and if I remember correctly, my personal best was 25 laps of the corridor in five minutes. Mo Farah would be impressed.

As my legs were getting all the exercise, I spoke to the Physiotherapist to find out if he had any equipment that I could use from my bed. He came back with a long blue wide elastic TheraBand resistance band and gave me an impressive demonstration on the variety of exercises I could use it for, whilst in bed. This included hooking the middle of the band underneath both feet, holding one end of the band in each hand and pulling the bands towards my chest. It was essentially a dumbbell bicep curl, laying down. He showed me many variations that could benefit the muscles in the arms, chest and stomach. One of my favourites was to loop the band around the metal bar at the end of the bed, hold one end of the band in each hand and use it in the movement of a rowing machine. This meant I was working my arms, legs, stomach and strengthening my core muscles. For more of a challenge, I just looped the end of the band around my hand another time, making the band shorter and, therefore, increasing the level of resistance.

The reason I am sharing this with you, is that a TheraBand can be used in the comfort of your own home, when seated, or in bed, or standing. As previously covered in Chapter 12 Healthy Lifestyle the British Lymphology Society and NHS both endorse and encourage regular movement for people with lymphoedema. TheraBands are not that expensive to buy, (Amazon: £2.85-£15) and you can tailor the level of resistance to suit your level of strength. As you would expect, there are many videos on YouTube demonstrating various exercises using the band.

There are many listed on Amazon, but this one caught my eye. OMERIL Resistance Bands Set of 3, Skin-Friendly Exercise Bands for £9.08 (usually £12.99) excluding postage. It includes a carry bag and user manual. There are other brands available, naturally.

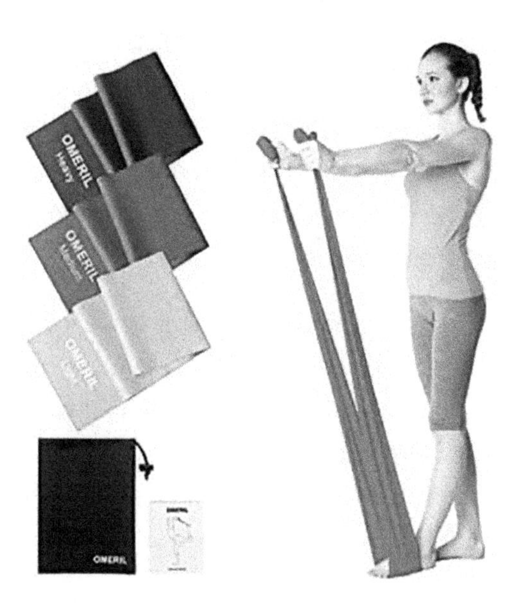

OMERIL Resistance Bands

Top Tip #39: Purchase a TheraBand and use it as part of your daily movement and exercise, in the comfort of your own home. Check out YouTube for instructional videos.

I am in no doubt that these exercises, walking the laps every hour, plus the numerous flights of stairs, positively contributed to my preparation for liposuction surgery. I did as much as I could do to put myself in the best possible position, both physically and mentally, to play my part in making this procedure as successful as possible.

On the 14th January, it was Hope's birthday, the first nurse I'd met from the wonderful nursing team who looked after me so well during my two-week stay. I spoke with the Ward Sister and hatched a plan. In usual hospital patient attire of shorts, t-shirt, dressing gown, slippers, plus numerous rolls of bandages wrapped around my entire leg, I headed downstairs to M&S

and bought a birthday card, cake and candles. Later that day, the Ward Sister, the nursing team and I hid in a darkened staffroom with the candles burning on a large chocolate birthday cake. A nurse told Hope that she was wanted in the staffroom and when she appeared, we all cheered and sang Happy Birthday to her. Her beautiful beaming smile got even bigger with her surprise, which was absolutely priceless.

I think that had the effect of lifting their spirits. My early observations that week had made me realise and appreciate that this was a particularly challenging ward to work in. Sadly, most of the patients had dementia or Alzheimer's disease, which was heart-breaking to see and opened my eyes to how lucky I was, actually. It put a lot of things into perspective for me, that's for certain.

The following day, 15th January 2017, was my 46th birthday and after five days in hospital I had a steady flow of visitors including my parents, sister and brother-in-law, my niece and nephew and of course, my wife and youngest daughter. My eldest daughter had to attend a funeral so couldn't make it. It was wonderful to see everyone, especially on my birthday. Not to be outdone, Hope had also hatched a plan. During a gap in visitors, one by one Hope and the other nurses gathered around the end of my bed with big smiles, before breaking into a rendition of "Happy Birthday to you". Bless them! But that wasn't all. Hope then presented me with a huge sponge cake with lashings of fresh cream and strawberries, in addition to a card and a gift. Amazing! I was grateful to be on this ward, cared for by these tremendous nurses and I felt overwhelmed by their efforts. I will never forget them and the difficult job that they do in this often traumatic ward.

Just a quick side-story if I may, and there are many I could tell you about my stay in St George's. I was in a bay of six beds, all full, with five other patients either suffering from dementia or Alzheimer's disease, which was incredibly sad to see. The patient opposite me was an elderly Irish gentleman, who was in a bad way. It transpired that a couple of months prior, he was fit and well and, whilst at a wedding, he had fallen down some steps and banged his head. Not long after returning home, he started to show signs of dementia and was admitted to hospital a few weeks before I arrived. He was terribly thin and had refused to eat anything for a couple of days. I tried to talk to him, asking what his favourite meal was. His quiet, mumbled response was an Irish Breakfast. We agreed that if I could get the hospital kitchen to make this for him, that he would try to eat it. I walked to the main hospital restaurant and spoke to the chef, who was fabulous. After I explained the situation, the team did their very best to produce as close to an Irish Breakfast as possible. I carried this back to the ward triumphant in the hope that my roommate would be tempted. Unfortunately, the smell of a freshly cooked breakfast wasn't appealing enough, and he didn't manage a single bite. A couple of days later he sadly passed away. Being on this ward gave me a huge realisation of how lucky I am, 'only' having lymphoedema. Don't get me wrong, it's been challenging as you have read, but at least it wouldn't kill me. During my two weeks in Amyand Ward, a further two patients lost their battles and died. This had been a truly humbling experience witnessing the fragility of the brain, and the fragility of life.

Moving on to the day of the surgery, I was very excited indeed. The intensive bandaging, exercise (movement) and healthy eating (plus no booze for two months) had paid off and my leg looked the best it had, ever! Did I actually need surgery? I was happy with the results so far, but deep down I knew that without surgery, the volume in my leg would soon rebound as it had so many times before.

I was taken down to the Day Surgery Unit and shown to the waiting room. Ms Milroy came to see me to run through the plan. It wasn't too long before I was taken into theatre and prepped for the anaesthetic and surgery. My mood was positive and jovial. I was certain that today would be the start of the journey to get my life back to where I needed it to be, for so many reasons.

When I woke up in recovery, the first thing I remember is the unbearable pain across the top of my foot. My leg was fully bandaged in Multi-Layer Lymphoedema Bandaging (MLLB). My requests to loosen the bandaging around the foot were soon agreed to, but unfortunately it was not enough to prevent the pain. Remarkably, that was the only pain I experienced post-surgery and throughout the whole recovery process.

I was taken back to the ward and around 24 hours later, Mark Pearson, an experienced Lymphoedema Therapist who I'd known for many years, came to my bedside to take off the bandages, check and clean up the leg, before reapplying the MLLB again. It was at this point, we noticed two things. The first was the absolutely staggering and unbelievable reduction in the size of my left leg, quite beyond anything I had imagined or hoped for. The second thing was the start of a pressure ulcer on the top of my foot. A picture tells a thousand words. So, here are photos of my legs taken in 2011 on the left, and again in July 2017 as a result of liposuction surgery on the right.

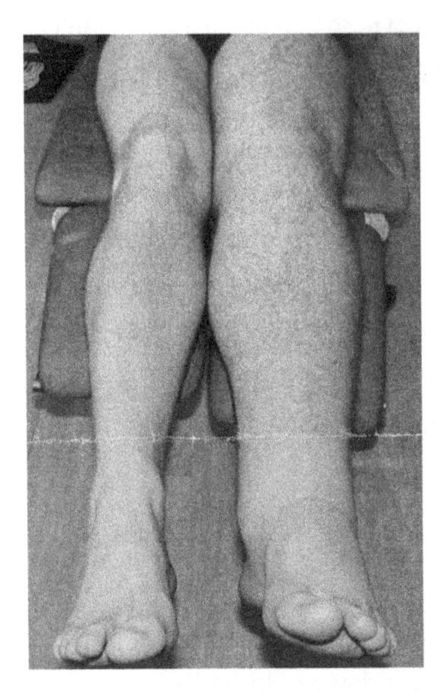

Matt's lymphoedema in 2011: pre-treatment

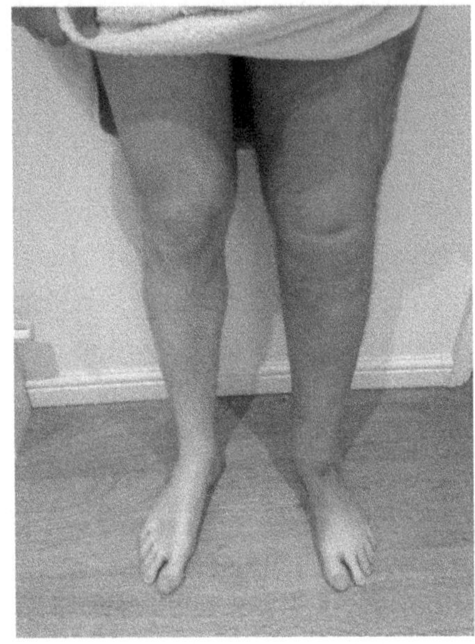

Matt's lymphoedema Autumn 2017: post-liposuction

As you can see, for me the liposuction surgery itself, was a tremendous success. Ms Milroy removed over two litres of fatty tissue from my lower leg alone, which took her around four hours. She must have been exhausted!

As my lower leg took so much time, she decided (as I was pre-warned) that the thigh would have to be done at a later date.

During week two, post-surgery, the nurses looked after me incredibly well and there was a constant flow of visits from many different medical professionals including: Professor Mortimer, Ms Milroy, Dr Gordon, Patryk Gawrysiak, practically all the lymphoedema therapists and several medical students. During the week, my wife and daughter visited again, (a four-hour round trip), along with my parents and two of my best friends. I was kept busy with these visits, daily MLLB treatment, and regularly having my obs done by the nurses. In between, I would exercise and walk laps of the corridor. I have to say, the bruising was spectacular and lasted several weeks but, amazingly, still no pain.

A week later, on my final day before discharge, a therapist helped me to put on my new class 4S compression made-to-measure stocking. She then gave me a new appropriately sized easywrap compression system to use at home. Shortly, after 14 days in hospital, I was packing my bag ready to return home with a much thinner leg, in the hope of getting my life back on track again. The outcome of this surgery was life-changing in so many ways.

Measurements taken in July 2018 showed a volume reduction of an unbelievable 17% larger than the right leg. In this meeting, Dr Gordon and Ms Milroy examined my leg and deemed me suitable for round two of liposuction surgery, subject to the CCG approving funding, of course.

Almost to the day, two years later in January 2019, I was back in the Amyand Ward of St George's Hospital to have the second phase of liposuction surgery, this time on my thigh. It was lovely seeing all the nurses again and a 'welcome back' hug from Hope. Knowing what to expect, I soon settled back into my routine, stocked up supplies from M&S, before my first session of MLLB. Once the bandages were on, I would restart my hourly exercises including, yes, walking laps of the corridor and the many flights of stairs, every hour, on the hour.

During my two-week stay, I met a gentleman in the ward, whilst on my way back from a walk. He was also having MLLB, on both legs and, it is fair to say, he looked like he was struggling a bit. I introduced myself and we had a lengthy conversation about lymphoedema, swapping tips on how we best manage the condition. He was having liposuction for the first time and I was able to answer many of his questions as I'd had this surgery before.

His main frustration was the struggle of being mobile with both of his legs in bandaging. Over the next day or so we had further conversations and I encouraged him to sign up as a member of the LSN to obtain information and advice. He was also curious about my hourly exits from the ward. Once I had explained the importance of movement, especially as part of MLLB treatment, he became more determined to try and increase his level of movement.

It wasn't too long before he was out of bed and walking downstairs and across to the main entrance shops, every day thereafter. Fellow lymphoedema sufferer, if you are reading this, I really hope that you are doing well. If you would like to get in touch with me, please send a message via my website *www.lymphoedemaunited.com* or email *matt@lymphunited.com*. I would be very interested to know how you are getting on.

On the day of surgery and knowing the process well, I was once again excited for the liposuction to proceed and for Ms Milroy to perform her miracles. She removed over one litre of fat from my thigh and, once again, liposuction had been a huge success for me. When I came around from the anaesthetic, the MLLB bandaging used in 2017 had been swapped for the easywrap Velcro compression system. This gave me more control to adjust the level of compression if required.

The recovery phase went tremendously smoothly both during the week in hospital, and for the following weeks recuperating at home. All was good in the world and my leg looked, well, fantastic, even if I do say so myself. These photos were taken post-surgery, whilst in hospital, inbetween daily MLLB treatment.

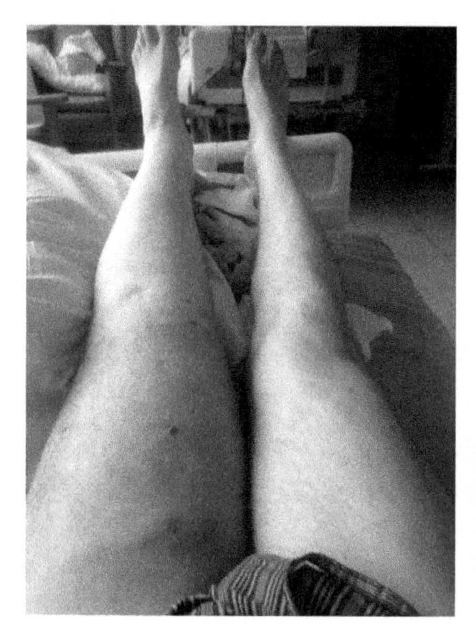

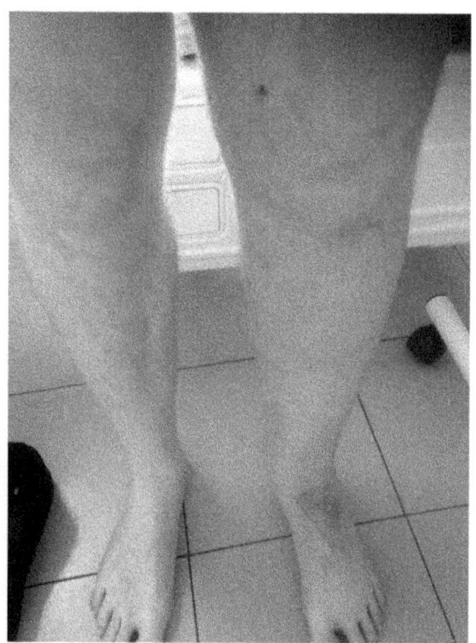

Matt's legs January 2019 – shortly after his second liposuction surgery

I would like to take this opportunity to sincerely thank Professor Peter Mortimer, Dr Kristiana Gordon, Ms Catherine Milroy, Carmen Chang, Patryk Gawrysiak, Mark Pearson and the team of lymphoedema therapists, plus all the nurses on the Amyand Ward, with a special mention to Hope. I am so grateful for your care, diligence and time spent with me during this life-changing procedure. *Excluding* the remarkable reduction in fluid through DLT, liposuction surgery removed over three litres of fatty tissue from my leg (equivalent to 3kg in weight). I would never have imagined this level of volume reduction was possible. Thank you all for your individual contribution, specifically during this remarkable two-year period of my life.

21

LYMPHATICS AND THE IMMUNE SYSTEM

"The coronavirus pandemic and vaccination efforts have brought the importance of a properly functioning lymphatic system into sharper focus."

—Dr Julian Pearce MBChB,
BSc (Hons) MRCP

A subject that prompted my interest, especially during the Covid-19 pandemic, was the important role that the lymphatics have with the immune system. Quite frankly this had not been on my radar at all until I read a book by Gemma Levine called Covid Thoughts. I met Gemma a few years ago when I was a case study in Gemma's book with Professor Mortimer called "Let's Talk Lymphoedema". As Gemma is a prolific author, I spoke with her to glean some tips before I started writing this book. That's when I ordered both of her books Covid Thoughts and Aqua, on sale on the St George's Hospital Charity online shop.

As with my book, Gemma's books are also raising money for the Lymphoedema Research Fund. Buy your copy here: *www.stgeorgeshospitalcharity.org.uk/shop/covid-thoughts*.

One of the first pages in Covid Thoughts that grabbed my attention, was the Foreword written by Professor Peter Mortimer. Without giving too much away and preventing you from buying Gemma's book, he starts by saying:

"Long term acquired Immunity from Covid infection requires a working lymphatic system."

"For the vaccine to work against Covid, a functional lymphatic system is essential" followed by

"The above two statements illustrate the importance of the lymphatic system for our immunity and for the fight against Covid."

To find out more, you'll have to buy the book and, in doing so, raise money for the Lymphoedema Research Fund.

When I discussed this further with Professor Mortimer, he suggested I speak with Dr Julian Pearce to ask if he would write about this very important subject in my book. I did just that and I am very grateful that he agreed. Dr Julian Pearce is a Dermatology Registrar and Academic Clinical Fellow at St. George's Hospital, London.

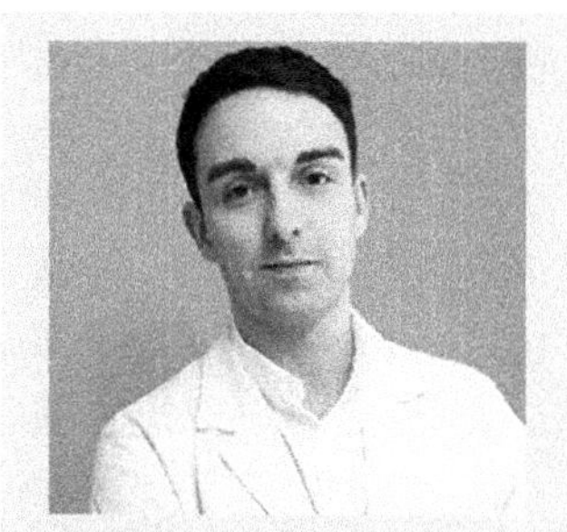

Dr Julian Pearce MBChB, BSc (Hons) MRCP
Dermatology Registrar and Academic Clinical Fellow

Matt and I were introduced by Professor Peter Mortimer, who kindly suggested I write a chapter for this book addressing the link between the lymphatic and immune systems. Professor Mortimer and I both work within the dermatology and lymphoedema department at St George's Hospital, London and are part of the lymphoedema research team at St George's, University of London.

Why your lymphatics are important for your immune system

The immune system is a complex concept which many patients (and doctors!) struggle to fully understand. A helpful parallel is to compare its components to an army fighting a war. The soldiers represent the immune cells, such as B and T lymphocytes, which work to patrol the body for invaders and fight infection. The soldiers travel within lymph through the lymphatic vessels which are present all throughout the body and set up camp at strategically placed lymph nodes in the neck, under-arms and groin. Invaders such as bacteria and viruses are absorbed by lymph vessels, and their presence trigger the soldiers into action, sending messages to one other, warning of the attack and packing into lymph nodes to adapt and arm themselves with the necessary resources to fight effectively. During an infection, the lymph nodes can therefore swell with an expanding artillery of fighters, explaining why we can sometimes feel them enlarge when unwell. Once fully armed and readied for battle, the soldiers then travel back through the lymphatics to the site of invasion and kill the assailants, protecting the body.

One can therefore appreciate that the lymphatic and immune systems are inherently interconnected. They develop together in the embryo and mature after we are born, working synchronously to adapt and protect us from threats such as infection.

So, what impact does lymphoedema have on our immune system, and vice versa? Our understanding is currently limited, mainly due to very little research in this area. This may seem surprising, based upon our observations above. Only recently has science begun to appreciate this link and I predict our knowledge will significantly improve in the coming years.

There is emerging evidence that some forms of genetically related lymphoedema are associated with a measurable reduction in circulating immune cells in the blood. The significance of reduced immune cell numbers in the blood is largely unknown at present, but the vast majority of patients do not seem to be at significantly higher risk of contracting communicable diseases such as the flu virus or COVID-19. It maybe that the immune cells are actually elsewhere, such as being trapped within the swollen areas of the body, rather than being measurable in the blood, or are lost through the gut if patients have a more widespread lymphatic problem. It may be that the genetic cause of their lymphoedema is also causing fewer immune cells to be produced. More research into these theories will inevitably improve our understanding of the interaction between genetics, the lymphatic and immune systems.

It has been known for some time that areas affected by lymphoedema are vulnerable to infection, whether genetically related or acquired, for example after cancer treatment. This will be familiar to many patients who suffer from recurrent, often severe, skin infections related to their swelling such as cellulitis where bacteria enter through small breaks in the skin, causing infection. This manifests as a localised redness, discomfort, warmth and worsening of the swelling.

Infection of skin affected by lymphoedema will require longer courses of antibiotics, compared to patients without lymphoedema, something many doctors may not appreciate. There are very helpful cellulitis guidelines (link at the end of this chapter) which patients can flag to their doctor, to help ensure the correct treatment is given for an appropriate duration. If patients are having more than two episodes of cellulitis per year requiring antibiotics, doctors may advise starting preventative (prophylactic) antibiotics to help prevent this. Other common infections include viral warts, which can also be very stubborn to treat. The difficulty in treating these infections is likely due the difficulty faced by the immune soldiers moving into, through and out of the damaged and congested lymph vessels.

What can be disheartening is that cellulitis can also damage the lymphatic vessels themselves. The bacteria and immune cells release destructive substances which can affect the integrity of the lymphatic vessel walls. Recurrent cellulitis can therefore lead to a vicious cycle, with the area affected by lymphoedema already being vulnerable to infection, with the infection worsening swelling, increasing the possibility of further infection.

However! There are definitely simple and effective steps which can be taken by patients and their doctors to reduce the risk of local infections and treat them appropriately, please see my 'top tips' below!

The coronavirus pandemic and vaccination efforts have brought the importance of a properly functioning lymphatic system into sharper focus.

Vaccines contain small, harmless parts of the bacteria or viruses which they aim to protect against. Once injected, your immune cells prime themselves to identity, target and destroy the invader should they encounter it again. The lymphatic vessels are the vital channels through which the vaccine contents and immune cells travel, and the lymph nodes are where the majority of your long-lasting immunity develops.

It is important to briefly discuss COVID-19 due to the current global pandemic at the time of writing. The vast majority of patients with lymphoedema will not be at increased risk from COVID-19. However, there are a few points worth mentioning regarding vaccination against this virus, and in general. Firstly, as we have seen the areas of lymphoedema are vulnerable to infection. Therefore, a needle piercing the skin in these areas could lead to a portal of entry for infection. Secondly, immune cells likely find it difficult to navigate their way into, through and out of the lymphatic vessels in areas affected by lymphoedema. For vaccination to be as effective as possible, the injection should ideally be into a limb or buttock unaffected by lymphoedema, or an area chosen which is least affected by swelling. We have produced a helpful document (link at the end of this chapter) to help guide patients and doctors with decisions such as these regarding vaccination.

I hope that this chapter has highlighted the important links between the lymphatic and immune systems. There is still much we don't know, but research and interest within this area is growing! The more we can learn about the interplay between these two complex and vital systems, the more we can truly understand about lymphoedema and the possibility of better, more effective treatments.

Top Treatment Tips!

1. Keep your skin well moisturised. This will maintain the skin barrier and reduce the risk of microbes entering the skin and causing infection
2. Optimise your compression. The greater the swelling the more at risk the skin is of local infection
3. Recognise the signs of cellulitis early so that you can obtain prompt treatment from your doctor
4. Take at least two weeks of antibiotics for cellulitis. Don't be nervous to signpost the 'cellulitis in lymphoedema' guidelines to your doctor!

Further helpful resources:

1 Cellulitis guidance: *https://www.lymphoedema.org/wp-content/uploads/2020/01/cellulitis_consensus.pdf*

2 COVID vaccination guidance: *https://www.lymphoedema.org/wp-content/uploads/2021/02/Consensus_Document_on_COVID_Vaccination_12feb2021.pdf*

22

GLOBAL AWARENESS: LYMPH IN THE USA

"The speed with which we succeed in finding those cures depends on the lymphatic community."

—William Repicci, President & CEO of Lymphatic Education & Research Network

In Chapter 5, Finding the Right Kind of Therapist, I wrote briefly about the Centers of Excellence created by the Lymphatic Education & Research Network (LE&RN). Taken from their website, "*LE&RN provide a geographically diverse network of multidisciplinary clinical care and service Centers for individuals and families affected by Lymphatic Diseases (LD). In addition to clinical and social services, the Centers provide professional and lay education in the geographic areas they serve, are involved in LD clinical research and work with LE&RN locally and internationally in its efforts to continually improve the lives of those, and their families, affected by Lymphatic Disease.*"

I have been exchanging many emails with William Repicci during 2021 and I am confident that we will work together again on other projects in the very near future.

I was very happy to purchase tickets and attend online, the LE&RN Virtual Global Celebration honouring World Lymphoedema Day on 6th March 2021, hosted by their spokesperson and award-winning Hollywood actor, Kathy Bates. The online event also featured the debut performance of the one-act play *Let's Talk Lymphedema* by Brian Daniels, based on the book written by Professor Peter Mortimer and Gemma Levine. LE&RN Honorary Board Member and actor Steve Guttenberg (Police Academy and Three Men and a Baby) performed the role of Professor Pembleton. No prizes for guessing who that character was based on!

I was a case study in this book, but I didn't even get through to the auditions on this occasion. More acting lessons required in time for the sequel perhaps!

The whole event was an enjoyable watch and a very welcomed break from the norm, especially during the third Covid-19 lockdown! Being online, the event was able to attract a global audience, importantly raising awareness of lymphedema (as spelt in the USA) and lymphatic disease (LD).

I asked what developments there had been with our lymphoedema allies across the pond? William was very happy to tell us.

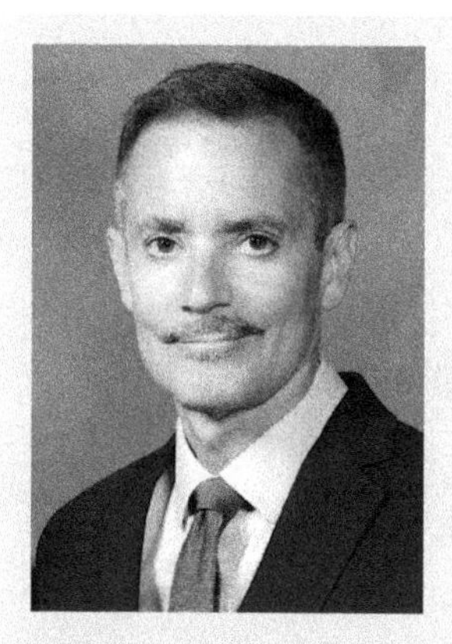

William Repicci
President & CEO
Lymphatic Education & Research Network (LE&RN)

I thank my friend and colleague, Professor Peter Mortimer, for introducing me to Matt Hazledine in early 2021. Since then, Matt and I have been involved in a torrent of emails fuelled by his determination to be a game-changer in this quickly evolving field of lymphatic disease (LD). The fact that Matt lives with lymphedema (LE) was of particular interest to me. I am always looking for the leaders who will forge the changes needed before LDs and LE become global priorities. Those leaders need to be activists who live with these diseases. Only those with the most at stake can commandeer the ears of powerbrokers who control the resources we need for future treatments and cures. And only leaders with LDs will arouse the passions of the lymphatic community as they evolve into activists. Matt and I began our conversation by grappling with issues such as the need for easily remembered acronyms, to the power of language in describing LE as either a "condition" or a "disease." The bond that ensued from our likeminded curiosity and determination led to Matt asking me to write a chapter for this book. I do so with pleasure and as prologue to what I envision as Matt's future impact on this field.

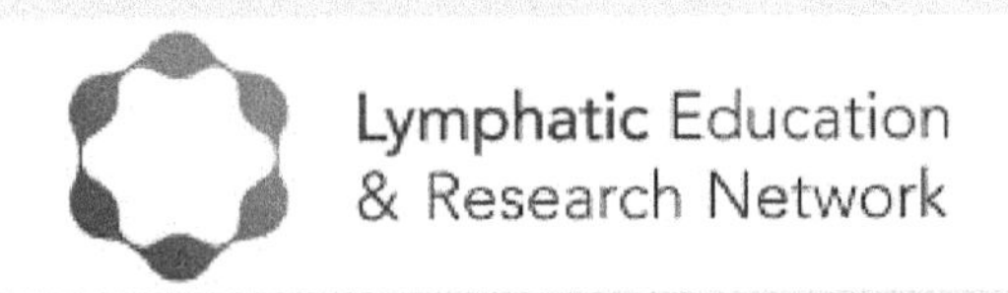

The Road to Cures Through Lymphedema and Lymphatic Disease Activism

There is a simple truism that drives the Lymphatic Education & Research Network (LE&RN): Activism=Research=Cures. Everything we do supports this axiom. The speed with which we succeed in finding those cures depends on the lymphatic community. AIDS went from an unknown fatal disease, to a world-recognized and treatable one in 25 years. This success took the unrelenting lobbying of advocates who would not accept "no" for an answer from governments, foundations, or potential donors. One was either on the front lines, or complicit in the death of those they loved. The AIDS campaign's motto was both succinct and direct: Silence=Death. The stakes were clear. It would then take billions of research dollars to realize their goal. According to UNAIDS, there are 38 million people worldwide living with HIV/AIDS. The World Health Organization estimates that 250 million globally live with lymphedema (LE).

No two causes are identical, but we can appreciate similarities among campaigns and the lessons to be learned. There is nothing new about LE. There are ancient carvings in India and Egypt depicting the disease. Yet, it is very likely that most people who have LE will go undiagnosed and untreated for many years. It is equally as likely that when they discover they have LE, the pervading general lack of awareness about the disease will have them thinking they are the only ones in the world with it. For those with LE related to cancer treatment, it is common that they have been told they should be grateful to be alive, find a therapist, and refrain from complaining. The result is that people living with LE feel isolated and alone as they face an incurable, debilitating, disfiguring disease that leaves them prone to infection while being psychosocially bruised. Well-meaning family, friends, and caretakers compound the anxiety of those living with LE by underplaying their suffering. Professionals are often heard to mitigate the impact of LE by stating that one doesn't die from the disease. However, this is disingenuous. People living with LE do die from the side effects. Antibiotics commonly fail to reverse the toll of infections, and associated obesity and lack of mobility play their own role in shortening life-expectancy. However, merely noting the loss of quality of life caused by this disease is more than enough to justify a call to action. To grow an activist movement, we must first dismantle prevailing constructs that hold back progress. With a mission to fight lymphedema and lymphatic diseases through education, research and advocacy, LE&RN has been endeavoring to do just this since its founding in 1998.

LE&RN's education efforts include funding Lymphedema Therapist Scholarships, monthly livestream symposiums by world leaders, a robust website with a multitude of downloadable resources and articles, the establishing of World Lymphedema Day on March 6th as a global day of celebration and activism, and the establishing of Chapters worldwide where people with lymphatic disease can connect, find support, and drive change in their communities. It also means getting the word about lymphedema into the broader community. As such, LE&RN has pursued celebrity ambassadors who support our cause, such as Dame Judi Dench, Steve Guttenberg and Wendy Williams. LE&RN also has a Global Spokesperson in Academy Award winner Kathy Bates. As LE&RN's Spokesperson, Ms. Bates, who has LE, has tirelessly taken our cause to innumerable conferences, television shows, magazine interviews, and Congressional legislative meetings. All these efforts are meant to further our goal of making lymphedema part of the global conversation. Before we garner the public's support to fund and find a cure, they first must know the disease's name and what is at stake.

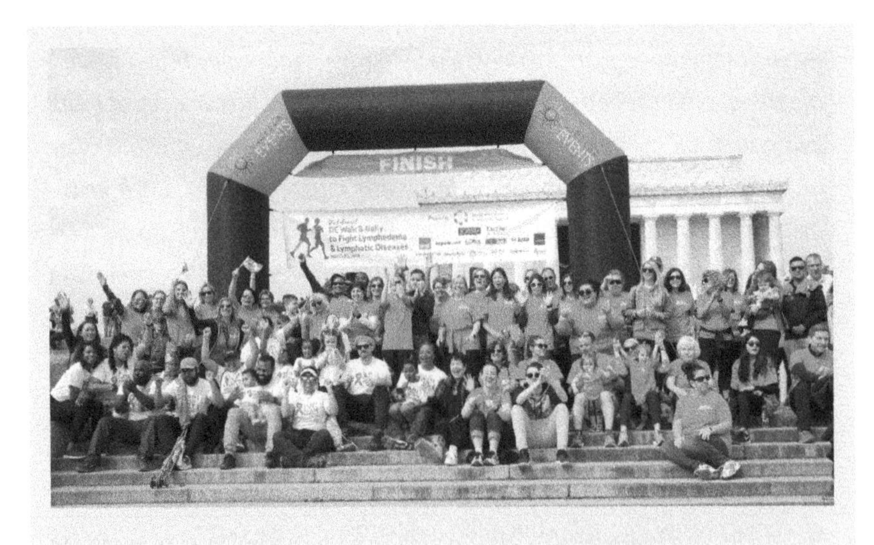

LE&RN 2019 - DC Rally at The Lincoln Memomorial

To foster research, LE&RN awards fellowships and scholarships to support the best and brightest researchers into our field. We organize and partner with several lymphatic conferences and publish the only peer-review journal in lymphatics, Lymphatic Research & Biology. We created The International Lymphatic Disease and Lymphedema Patient Registry and Biorepository so that researchers have access to the data they need for tomorrow's breakthroughs. Research requires funding and, as such, LE&RN lobbies the United States legislature, the National Institutes of Health, the Department of Defense and the Centers of Disease Control and Prevention to focus research dollars on lymphatics. To educate medical practitioners, LE&RN creates online continuing medical education courses for physicians. To guarantee that people living with lymphatic diseases can find medical care, LE&RN established the first worldwide standards for Centers of Excellence in the Diagnosis and Treatment of Lymphatic Diseases. After a rigorous review process by a global oversight committee chaired by Prof. Peter Mortimer of St. George's University Hospital, London, and Melissa Aldrich, PhD of UT Health, USA, we award this status to institutions that will provide all-encompassing and state-of-the-art care to those living with lymphatic diseases. At the time of writing this article, there are 25 Centers of Excellence globally with another 20 institutions with applications under evaluation. This reveals a sea-change in the future of care for lymphatic diseases.

Once we have an informed public and an invested research community, our attention turns to advocacy. There are many ways that one can get LE. Beyond those with genetic, hereditary, or acquired LE from cancer treatment, surgery, physical trauma or bacterial infection, there are those with LE related to lymphatic filariasis and podoconiosis. No matter how one develops this disease, we are one family and need to join in one fight. To galvanize this support, each year LE&RN petitions the World Health Organization to make lymphedema their focus.

Along with researchers and practitioners, the LE community needs to invest themselves in this cause. Funding entities would be hard-pressed to deny 250 million people who demand change. Change will not come by waiting for others to fight one's battle. Change will not come if the community sits in silence and hides their disease. Change will be difficult to come by if people with LE continue to speak about the disease as a mild "condition" instead of acknowledging it as a debilitating and progressive disease. Change will occur when those living with LE, and all those who care about them, stand up and loudly state that this devastating disease must be cured. Every country needs to be contributing research funding to this end. It is up to the LE/LD community to drive this point to a successful conclusion.

We live at a time when the future is so very promising. Clinical research is growing at an exponential rate. Lymphatic related drug trials, new surgeries, and innovative diagnostic equipment are rapidly changing the field. We now hear about therapeutic strategies with the potential to lessen and even prevent LE. Hope abounds. The good news is that the speed at which we succeed is entirely in our hands. This leaves only one question for everyone reading this article: "Am I ready to dedicate myself to this cause until we win this war against lymphedema and lymphatic diseases?"

If the answer to this question is yes, then visit the LE&RN website for further information or to make contact www.lymphaticnetwork.org.

Thank you, William. I cannot wait to meet you in person to discuss how we can collaborate and continue our mission to increase awareness, raise money for research and help others to live better with lymphoedema, or lymphedema as you would say.

23

RAISING GLOBAL AWARENESS & HELPING OTHERS WORLDWIDE

"I wonder what else could be achieved if we all pulled together to help others around the world to live better with lymphoedema?"

—Matt Hazledine,
Author and Managing Director of Lymphoedema United

I think that it's a very fair assumption to make, that the vast majority of human beings are good people and at some stage in their life have tried to help others less fortunate than themselves. Whether that's donating or raising money for a well-known charity like Cancer Research or NSPCC or pledging money during a telethon by Comic Relief or Children in Need. Of course, it doesn't have to be financial to make a difference. Giving unwanted clothes and possessions to the local charity shops such as The British Red Cross or looking after an elderly or vulnerable neighbour can be as, if not more, effective. I believe that helping others in their time of need is in our genetic make-up.

In Chapter 4 How Common is Chronic Oedema, Professor Christine Moffatt wrote "*Lymphoedema affects approximately 250 million people worldwide*[2] *with 120 million people being affected by a neglected tropical disease Lymphatic Filariasis, a type of lymphoedema caused by a mosquito bite. Lymphatic Filariasis occurs mainly in India and Africa and causes mainly genital lymphoedema in men (25 million) and elephantiasis of the leg in women mostly (15 million)*[3]*. In fact we do not know how many people are affected by Chronic Oedema in the world because of the many different conditions associated with it.*"

We have all no doubt, used the old saying at some point in our life *"There's always someone else worse off than me".* Whether that person is in our town, county, country or world, there are those who put their own ailments aside to help others, regardless of whether they know them or not.

Over many decades, the media has publicised all too regular footage of poorer countries struggling to control the spread of diseases, resulting in millions of untimely deaths. I grew up as a child of the 80s and remember vividly the news reports about the famine in Ethiopia and other parts of Africa. This cause motivated Sir Bob Geldof and Midge Ure to take action and bring together the British and Irish pop royalty of the era, creating Band Aid to record the song "Do they know it's Christmas?". Released in 1984, the record alone is reported to have raised over £200m, with all the money raised going to charity. This then led to the historic concert, Live Aid, on 13th July 1985. This one-off event was viewed by an estimated audience of 1.9 billion people in 150 nations, accounting for nearly 40% of the world population, according to Wikipedia. According to *www.history.com* Live Aid concert raised $127 million for famine relief in Africa. It is also worth reminding ourselves that this took place before social media ever existed.

In January 2003, nearly 18 years after Live Aid, Greta Thunberg was born and was destined to become the young, passionate environmentalist activist from Sweden we all now know. By using social media effectively to get her unedited message across, Greta has demonstrated how, with a powerful message, we can quickly reach like-minded people, worldwide. Through social media, Greta has the portal to communicate directly with the world's population. She has attracted a staggering 4.9 million followers on Twitter (at the time of writing), no doubt all aligned with Greta's mission to help save our planet.

Often reported by the media as the "Greta Effect", her efforts have raised awareness of global climate change and encouraged us all to make changes in our lifestyle to reduce our carbon footprint and therefore, reduce carbon emissions. She is internationally known for challenging world leaders and is a force to be reckoned with, that's for sure. Is it perhaps no surprise that her parents named her Greta, an anagram of Great.

Sir Bob Geldof and Greta Thunberg are just two examples of people who have demonstrated what can be achieved if we all pull together to make a positive difference to help others from our wonderful and fragile planet.

Most recently, we have seen the horrendous loss of life caused by the Covid-19 global pandemic. At the time of writing this, The World Health Organisation (WHO) reports that up to 18th June 2021, there have been 176,945,596 confirmed cases of Covid-19, including 3,859,364 deaths globally. On the same date, the WHO reported that India had 29,700,313 confirmed cases and 381,903 deaths, but this is expected to increase further as the country is experiencing a catastrophic third wave of the virus. As wealthier countries, including the UK, are rapidly vaccinating their population, poorer or developing countries are not getting the vaccinations into the arms of their people in any such number. There have been many calls for the wealthier countries to provide vaccines to other countries struggling to contain the pandemic. After all, the virus travels and does not respect geographical borders. Unless we try to stop the global spread further, Covid will continue to kill millions more. This is one for the politicians worldwide and not one that, I dare say, even Sir Bob and Greta would struggle to solve.

So, bringing this back to the main subject of the book, how can we help others in the global lymphoedema community, especially those who are less fortunate than us, who perhaps do not have such a fabulous health care service as we do with the NHS in the UK?

With an estimated 250 million people in the world living with lymphoedema or chronic oedema, it would be satisfying for me to know that, when my time is up and I leave this earth, at least I had given it my best shot to help as many of these people as I possibly could.

As I have experienced too many times in my working life, there are the talkers and there are the doers. I know of people who have an unending flow of new ideas, but either lack ability or confidence to follow it through and make the idea a reality. Without blowing my own trumpet too loudly, when I have an idea that I think has mileage, I make it happen. Whether that's organising a charity golf day, setting up a new business, or writing a book and creating a new website, I will bring the idea to life.

However, I find more impact can be made when collaborating with other passionate, like-minded people. So, if you are interested in discussing ideas on how we can make a positive difference to the global lymphoedema community, please visit 'Contact Us' on my website and get in touch *www.lymphoedemaunited.com*.

In Chapter 9, The Importance of Properly Fitted Compression Garments, I asked you to give some thought to these two questions:

- What *do* you do with your old compression garments?
- What *could* you do with your old compression garments?

The reason I ask, is that for years I have held onto my old garments and stored them in a box or bag in the loft or garage. My hope was that I would find someone in the lymphoedema community who could put them to good use, perhaps by sending them to people struggling to control their lymphoedema in less privileged countries. I spoke to Professor Christine Moffatt CBE about this very subject during a recent video call. Unfortunately, my enthusiasm to add this project to my 'to do list' was dampened somewhat by Christine telling me that this had been investigated previously and was not found to be viable. She explained that the cost of shipping the garments abroad was more expensive than the actual cost to make the products in the first place, so the concept did not get off the ground.

I suppose the other element to consider supplying made-to-measure garments to other people, is whether they would be effective or not. As we read earlier, it is important to wear properly fitted compression garments. However, could it be more effective than not to wear any garment at all? As you would expect, I have tremendous respect for Professor Moffatt, and I can't wait to discuss this with her further in the near future.

Fortunately, I have fantastic relationships with many of the top medical experts who have been incredibly supportive of my projects. Professor Moffatt started telling me about the International Lymphoedema Framework (ILF), which is a dedicated platform for the lymphoedema community to improve the management of the condition and related disorders worldwide. I am very keen to find out more about the ILF and see if there is any way that I can help in some small way. For further information about the ILF, visit their website *www.lympho.org*.

I wonder what else could be achieved if we all pulled together to help others around the world to live better with lymphoedema?

24

A CURE? – RESEARCH & FUNDING

"Progress will only be made through research. Research brings scientific breakthroughs for new treatments which can be disseminated though education, which in turn feeds clinical practice and patient management."

—Professor Peter Mortimer MD, FRCP.
Professor of Dermatological Medicine

Since getting lymphoedema in 2011, I have tried pretty much anything and everything available to me, with the aim of reducing the size of my left leg to as close to 'normal' as possible.

The core objective of self-managing the condition has been to reduce the volume and, crucially, to maintain it. The fact of the matter is that my leg size is better, but the problem has not gone away. Am I resigned to the fact that lymphoedema is a chronic lifelong condition? The answer is probably yes, to be honest. I genuinely hope that there will be a ground-breaking cure to help future generations, through scientific and medical progress. At present, however, I am not convinced that lymphoedema is sufficiently visible on the Government's radar to command the attention it so rightly deserves. To find a cure, there first has to be medical research and the interest from scientists. I understand that for scientists to be interested in research, there has to be the funding in place to finance their work. How can a cure be found if there is a lack of funding, not enough interested scientists and, therefore, no research? Where is the funding coming from, the Government? Probably not, because of so much competition from other life-threatening diseases. Is the money coming from charitable donations, fundraising and legacies? Yes. Is this enough money initially to gain the interest from scientists? No. Is it sustainable to ensure the research continues to find a cure? Unlikely.

So, where is the money going to come from to support medical research? Are we ever going to find a cure for lymphoedema? I asked Professor Peter Mortimer, Professor of Dermatological Medicine, who is undeniably recognised as *the* most qualified and experienced 'go to' lymphoedema expert in the world.

I first met Professor Mortimer in February 2012 at St George's Hospital, London, in the hope that he would take me on as an NHS patient. Over nine years later I am still under the excellent care of the St George's team, with Dr Kristiana Gordon at the helm. I am proud to share with you, that I have truly excellent dialogue with Professor Mortimer and a relationship that has developed well beyond one typical of a medical professional and a patient, to one of mutual respect and friendship.

Regardless of the number of times he tells me of his plans to slow down and retire, Professor Mortimer remains in the thick of the action in the world of lymphoedema and probably will be for the foreseeable future. I was a case study in his book with Gemma Levine "Let's Talk Lymphoedema" (available on Amazon). In addition, he asked me to tell my story in the Good Health section in the Daily Mail back in May 2017, taking me right out of my comfort zone!

More recently, Professor Mortimer has been great support in being a sounding board for my new projects, has provided information and advice, as well as open some new doors for me. This has helped me tremendously in the process of writing this book and creating a new patient-orientated website which brings together people living with lymphoedema, medical professionals, organisations and specialist suppliers.

I am genuinely honoured to introduce you to Professor Peter Mortimer to answer the burning questions about the importance of funding to support scientific research which, in turn, may well lead to a cure for lymphoedema.

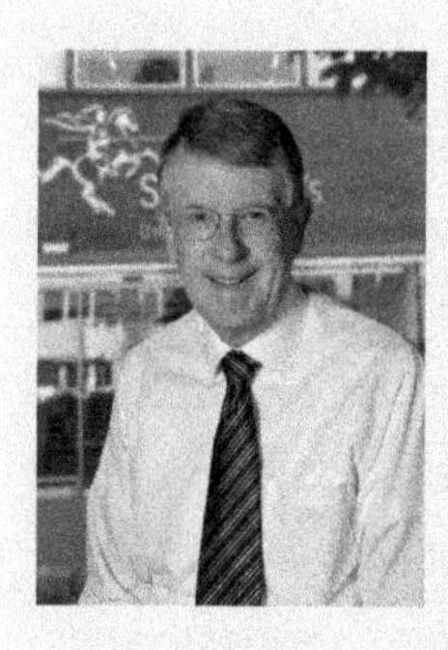

Peter Mortimer MD, FRCP
Professor of Dermatological Medicine
Molecular and Clinical Sciences Institute (Dermatology Unit)
St. George's, University of London and
Honorary Visiting Professor, Kings College, London

I have known Matt for almost ten years now and can honestly say, I regard him as a compliant patient with the drive to make a positive contribution by helping others with lymphoedema. In fact, during one of our consultation meetings at St George's Hospital in 2014, I suggested to Matt that he writes an article for the LSN Lymphline Newsletter to share his story and represent the male voice. He did just that and it was published in the Winter 2015 edition. The following year, Matt joined the Lymphoedema Support Network as a Trustee, which showed his commitment to the cause. Now, he is making new ground in creating this book, which I don't think has ever been done in this way before, as well as producing a new website, which again, I think provides a unique service to people living with lymphoedema. I am very pleased to have been Matt's sounding board, as he puts it, and provide him with support and encouragement along the way.

Matt knows that the subject of research is very important to me, as improvements in patient care can only come through research. That said, I am happy to answer his questions to the best of my knowledge, at the time of writing this book (April 2021): "Where is the money going to come from to support medical research?" and "Are we ever going to find a cure for lymphoedema?"

For generations, the UK has been a leading force in medical research and, once again, British scientists, this time at Oxford University, have shown the world the importance of research and funding in the rapid development, trials, testing and mass production of the Oxford University-AstraZeneca vaccine for Covid-19. This vaccine is being supplied globally to protect the human race from this uncompromising virus, responsible for over 2.7 million deaths worldwide, at the time of writing. From the time that the pandemic took a clenched grip of China, Europe, the UK, USA and the rest of the world, the race was on to produce the first effective vaccine. Sky News reported that Oxford University has received £65.5 million of funding from the Government's Vaccines Taskforce using public funds. This resulted in an effective vaccine being produced in a staggering ten months, injecting the arms of the most vulnerable British public, the first being Brian Pinker (aged 82) on 4th January 2021. This vaccine along with others including the Pfizer vaccine that was first given famously to Margaret Keenan (aged 91) on 8th December 2020, will go onto save an incomprehensible number of lives, that otherwise could have been lost to the Covid-19 disease.

The same comparison can be drawn with the disease that claimed so many lives around the world, in the 1980s. It is reported that 32.7 million lives have *been lost worldwide to AIDS caused by the Human Immunodeficiency Virus (HIV). Originally, HIV was said to have started in Africa and could be transmitted from person to person through blood and other bodily fluids, especially as a result of sharing syringes or through unprotected sex. Like all diseases, AIDS was not selective as to whom it infected. We lost Hollywood actor Rock Hudson and global rock star Freddie Mercury, amongst tens of millions of people who have lost their battle with AIDS. Since then, around $19-20 billion* ***every year****, has been invested in research to find a cure (source www.avert.org). At present, medical scientists have managed to produce medicine to manage the condition of HIV positive before it develops into AIDS, which, only too often, results in death.*

In both Covid-19 and HIV money was thrown to scientists and it worked. It worked because scientists thought the problems were important and the funding was available to do the research. The lymphatic system and the diseases with which it is thought to be involved i.e. lymphoedema are not considered important enough yet what is not commonly known is that for any ***vaccination*** *to work, it needs a working lymphatic system. That is because the vaccine has to get to the lymph nodes through transport by the lymphatic vessels for the immune cells of the body to be appropriately primed to provide the necessary immunity. Antibody production starts in the lymph nodes. Have you heard the lymphatic system mentioned during Covid-probably not!*

Turning to HIV and its relationship with lymphatic system, HIV is an infection of immune cells, particularly lymphocytes that live primarily in the lymphatic system. Most HIV is not in the blood but is lying deep within the body where most lymphocytes are located—in lymph nodes and lymphatic tissues. The human body can't get rid of HIV and no effective HIV cure exists. This is because HIV infected cells hide in the lymphatic system while HIV is undetectable in the blood. There is a desperate need to develop and test new anti-HIV therapies that can penetrate and be effective in lymphatic tissues. While HIV has received huge research funding, to find the cure scientists are going to have to know more about the lymphatic system.

Of course, there are many other well-known diseases that receive significant funding towards medical research, either from fundraising, donations or legacies. Cancer Research is arguably the most prominent in the UK. Their current advertising campaign (March 2021) states that one in two people will be affected by cancer in their lifetime, which does not fail to grab your attention. Cancer kills by spreading to other parts of the body. How does it do that? The answer is via the lymphatic system. Get the gist of my argument for supporting lymphatic research?

So, what about lymphoedema and other diseases of the lymphatic system? It is incredibly rare that one could die of lymphoedema, although not impossible due to the chance of getting sepsis as a result of cellulitis. It could happen. Therefore, given that lymphoedema doesn't cause death in the same numbers as Cancer, AIDS or Covid-19 do, to name a few, it is understandable that the level of funding received is practically non-existent in comparison. On the other hand, as covered several times during this book, lymphoedema is a chronic life-long disease which causes an enormous amount of suffering. Indeed, many patients express the view that their lymphoedema has been far more difficult to cope with than their cancer.

Professor William McMaster from Montreal was one of the first clinical scientists to demonstrate functioning skin lymphatic vessels using a novel technique involving the injection of a dye to visualise the lymphatics. He said in an oft-quoted Lecture of 1942: "The functions of the lymphatic system have remained largely unknown (since its discovery). Two influences have contributed to our state of ignorance, a lack of suitable methods of study . . . and a lack of interest". This statement still holds true today. To the lack of interest could be added a lack of research funding as difficulties in obtaining grants result in a lack of interest from scientists. It could be said that it was the availability of research funding that attracted scientists to move into the area of AIDS research. The greater number of scientists within a research field increase competition, and the output, and the breakthroughs.

Research needs money. The availability of funding drives research. Research discoveries feed education, which in turn feeds new treatments in clinical practice. Success breeds more interest and encourages further funding. It really is a vicious circle. Progress will only come from research when there is a critical mass of clinical and research scientists involved and interested in lymphoedema.

I am pleased to say that progress is being made in terms of our scientific understanding of what goes wrong with the lymphatic system. For example, in the genetic forms of primary lymphoedema and the discovery of the first causal gene of lymphoedema some 20 years ago, numerous other causal genes for lymphoedema have subsequently been discovered. Knowing the gene helps us to understand the mechanism of how a specific type of lymphoedema develops. This provides us with a target to aim for with regard to future new treatments.

Quite simply, more money is required to fund lymphatic research and attract the right medical scientists and doctors. This is a constant struggle in the lymphoedema sector, and it is equally difficult to attract more qualified therapists to the profession.

During the past 20 years, I have seen a considerable increase in the level of interest from scientists as more of them start to realise the importance of the lymphatic system not just to disease but to human health generally. One major problem for getting clinical doctors interested is that the lymphatic system features poorly in medical school curriculum teaching (because it has been traditionally considered unimportant). Therefore, the lymphatic system is not on the radar of doctors and, consequently, doctors do not recognise when they are confronted with a lymphatic disease. In the main, lymphoedema is not life-threatening and so considered a minor issue. Just because lymphoedema is not life-threatening, does not make it any less important as a disease, particularly as it can cause so much suffering. To try and address the issue of limited medical school teaching, we are developing a very specific lymphatic system learning module as part of the medical school curriculum at St George's University of London, so the medical students can be made aware about the lymphatic system and lymphatic diseases such as lymphoedema in the same way they learn about other diseases such as cancer and cardiovascular conditions.

Another major problem is that not one drug exists to treat a malfunctioning lymphatic system yet there are hundreds of drugs to treat a malfunctioning heart. Without the tools to treat a disease doctors are left helpless and disinterested.

Will a cure come from a drug? It has been widely documented that the anti-inflammatory drug Ketoprofen appeared to effectively treat lymphoedema symptoms and ease the burden of care, according to study results. (source www.healio.com/news/hematology-oncology on 1st Feb 2019). Stanley G. Rockson, MD, professor of cardiovascular medicine at Stanford University School of Medicine, said in a press release "Ketoprofen restores the health and elasticity of the skin. I believe it will reduce recurrent infection and can also reduce swelling. This new treatment does not cure lymphedema, but our studies show it has the capacity to make the illness more liveable and more workable." After working with animal trials 15 years earlier, the first exploratory trial included 21 human patients with primary or secondary lymphoedema received 75mg Ketoprofen three times daily. Researchers observed significant improvements in the inflammation and skin thickness at 4 months compared with baseline. However, the researchers reported that although there were no significant adverse events highlighted during the trial, they know that this class of nonsteroidal anti-inflammatory drugs is capable of causing significant side effects, such as gastrointestinal bleeding and effects on kidney function. It is doubtful that this drug will be produced as a treatment and not is it likely to provide a cure, but it is a start on that road to a solution.

As recently as March 2020, PureTech announced that the first participant had been dosed in a clinical study of LYT-100, the company's product candidate for the potential treatment of lymphoedema and other fibrotic conditions. LYT-100 is a selectively deuterated form of pirfenidone and has demonstrated anti-inflammatory and anti-fibrotic activity. Babak Mehrara, chief, plastic and reconstructive surgical service at Memorial Sloan Kettering Cancer Center, reported in www.pharmatimes.com/news "LYT-100 is designed to address the underlying cause of lymphoedema by reducing fibrosis and inflammation and restoring lymphatic function, and I believe it holds tremendous potential as a therapeutic candidate for the treatment of lymphoedema."

This is all very encouraging, but usually the creation, development, testing and approval of a new drug can usually take ten years before it is available to patients, unlike the Covid-19 vaccine which took ten months. The positive news is that progress is being made, albeit much slower than we would all like.

With increased knowledge of lymphatic science, born from research, one could argue that the lymphatic system is involved in some way in the majority of human diseases. A working lymphatic system is essential for overcoming infection, controlling body fluid balance, and for the absorption and metabolism of body fat. Furthermore, the lymphatic system is the main means by which cancer spreads and kills. We therefore need to improve further our understanding about how this very important system impacts on disease and how we can use that knowledge to develop new drug therapies. Hopefully then, doctors and scientists will become more aware and more interested.

We need more money available for lymphatic research to attract scientists into the sector. This was the main reason why I launched the Lymphoedema Research Fund in 2002. This fund is now under the care of The St George's Hospital Charity and Amerjit Chohan (Chief Executive Officer) will explain more about it in another chapter.

I was delighted when my patient and author, Matt Hazledine, approached me in January 2021 with the concept of his book and told me he will donate a percentage of profits to the Lymphoedema Research Fund. I am hopeful that the book will be a great success and raise lots of money for the fund.

Thank you very much to Professor Mortimer for providing the hope that, one day, a cure for lymphoedema may be found. If, sorry, *when* a cure is found, I'll be able to get my most favourite trousers and shoes back out of the 'spare' wardrobe again!! 😊

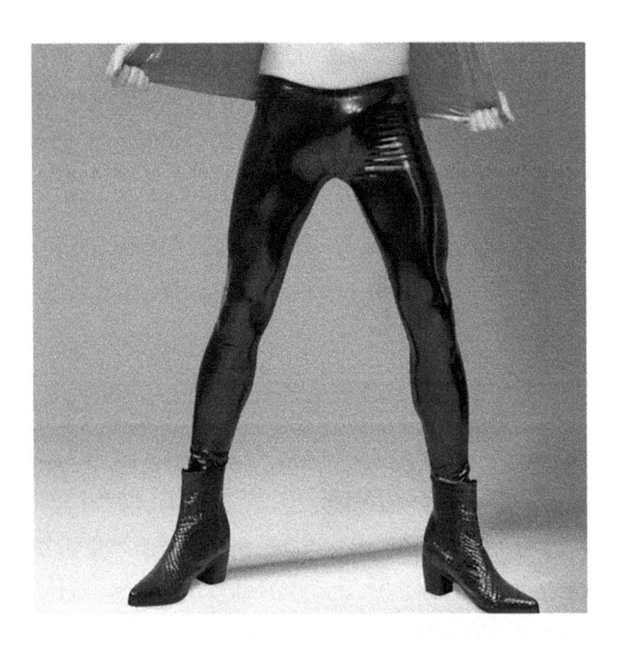

Bring on a cure and a return to 'normal' trousers again!

As Professor Mortimer says, there needs to be more money to attract scientists to conduct lymphatic research. That is, no doubt, why the Lymphoedema Research Fund was founded in the first place. Therefore, it falls on all of us with lymphoedema to help raise as much money as we can, or to donate an affordable amount (if budget allows) to the Research Fund. You have already made a start by purchasing this book, as I will explain in the next chapter.

Join me in the quest to fund research, so scientists can find a cure to help future generations to live better ***without*** lymphoedema.

25

ST GEORGE'S HOSPITAL CHARITY - LYMPHOEDEMA RESEARCH FUND

"St George's Hospital Charity is working hard to raise income to support and promote medical and scientific research focused primarily on lymphatics and the lymphatic system"

—Amerjit Chohan,
CEO, St George's Hospital Charity

When I spoke to Professor Mortimer in January 2021 about writing a book to pass on my experiences and tips to other people with lymphoedema, his reaction was very positive, and he provided lots of support and encouragement. The concept of the book quickly evolved with my idea of introducing medical professionals and experts, asking them to contribute to specific chapters.

During our initial conversation, we discussed the importance of funding and research to find a cure for lymphoedema. I could hear the passion and enthusiasm emanating from Professor Mortimer over the phone. He told me about the Lymphoedema Research Fund, which he set up as a registered charity in 2002, with the objective of raising money to fund research and find a cure. The obvious was staring me in the face and I committed there and then to use the book to raise money for this charity. As I am mostly self-funding this project, the intention has always been to cover my costs. Thereafter, I pledge to donate a minimum of 25% of pre-tax profits generated from the sales of this book to the Lymphoedema Research Fund.

After a lengthy telephone conversation with the CEO of the charity, I was convinced that raising money for this cause could benefit future generations of people to hopefully cure them of lymphoedema.

I was reassured that the Fund is there to generate money to support lymphatic research, to benefit everyone in the UK, and not just to support St George's Hospital.

To tell us more about the Lymphoedema Research Fund, which is now managed by The St George's Hospital Charity, allow me to introduce their CEO, Amerjit Chohan.

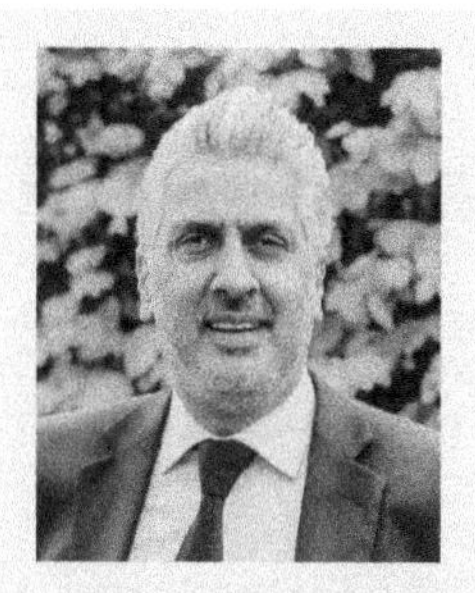

Amerjit Chohan
Chief Executive Officer
St George's Hospital Charity

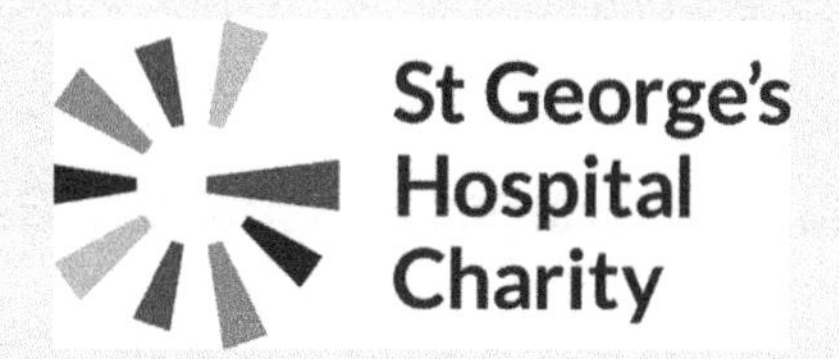

At St George's Hospital Charity our mission is to enhance the experience of patients, families, staff and the wider community served by St George's Trust. We are the official charity of St George's University NHS Foundation Trust.

The charity exists to support St George's and Queen Mary's hospitals and the communities they serve. We give grants and raise funds to improve the patient experience, improve facilities, support staff, provide equipment, enable ground-breaking research and fund an array of arts activities.

Every day, our work makes a real difference to patients, their families and friends and the staff who care for them.

OUR VISION AND MISSION

OUR VISION

Better care, healthier lives

OUR MISSION

We work to improve the experience of patients, families, staff and the wider community served by St George's hospitals.

OUR VALUES

- *We put patients first*
- *We are collaborative*
- *We make an impact*
- *We listen and respond*

Lymphoedema At St Georges Hospital & St George's University

St Georges Hospital is a tertiary referral national service providing expert assessment, diagnosis, treatment and continued support for those with lymphoedema. Patients with lymphoedema of all causes are treated, including primary lymphoedema (adults and children), and secondary to other problems (e.g. cancer-related lymphoedema, chronic venous oedema, lipoedema). The aim is to restore people with lymphoedema to as high a level of independence as is possible within the limits of their capabilities. Since lymphoedema is a chronic condition, the need to provide ongoing support is acknowledged.

Lymphoedema Research

St George's Hospital Charity is working hard to raise income to support and promote medical and scientific research focused primarily on lymphatics and the lymphatic system with a view to achieving advances in the prevention, diagnosis and treatment of lymphoedema and other disorders of the lymphatic system.

The charity aims to fund research that will focus on:

- *Supporting high quality medical and scientific research in which lymphatic biology and disorders of the lymphatic system are the main focus.*
- *Promoting interdisciplinary research that will result in advances in the prevention, diagnosis and treatment of lymphoedema and other lymphatic disorders.*
- *Providing funding for small and large scale clinical trials for possible improvements in treatment for patients with lymphoedema and other lymphatic disorders.*

With Your Support we aim to help the 200,000 plus people who suffer from lymphoedema and other disorders of the lymphatic system each year.

Please visit our website if you would like to know more about our work www.stgeorgeshospitalcharity.org.uk or email giving@stgeorges.nhs.uk if you would like to make a donation.

Thank You

We are incredibly grateful to Matt Hazledine who is donating 25% of the profits from this book to fund research into lymphoedema.

Matt's own personal journey with lymphoedema, (10 years in June 2021) gives him a clear understanding for the need to fund research.

Thank you Amerjit, for your passionate insight into the Lymphoedema Research Fund and St George's Hospital Charity.

Of course, there are many other worthwhile lymphoedema charities that need financial support, including the LSN, BLS and MLD^UK^, to name a few.

To use a well-known strapline from a major supermarket chain, "*Every Little Helps!*". Any money that you can afford to donate or generate through fund-raising to support these worthwhile charities, is much needed and gratefully received.

26

LYMPHOEDEMA UNITED AND LYMPHUNITED

During the first lockdown period of the Covid-19 pandemic in 2020, I started thinking about what I wanted to do with the rest of my working life. What was my passion? What was my purpose? What motivated me? Perhaps, coincidentally, my business partner at the time approached me with a proposal to buy my share of the business and the offices which we jointly owned. The timing was perfect for me and after a little negotiating, we agreed terms and I signed the contracts on 14th January 2021, the day before my 50th birthday. Coincidence or meant to be? I think the latter.

During 2019 and early 2020, pre-Covid-19, I was working one day per week as a consultant with Haddenham Healthcare on their new online patient shop, conveniently called LymphShop. The experience of working on this project, in addition to my time as a Trustee of the Lymphoedema Support Network, gave me the impetus and motivation to do something unique in this sector. I knew I was passionate about lymphoedema, but was it my purpose?

When I was first diagnosed with lymphoedema, the first few months were extremely daunting and isolating. I often compare it to wading through treacle in thick fog. I didn't know who or where to go to for help. I didn't know which products were most effective, so I bought anything and everything. I didn't want to talk about it and when I finally did, I didn't know who best to contact. I also didn't know, and neither did my GP, which experts I needed to be referred to.

This gave me the idea for what I needed then but didn't have, something that will help anyone who has lymphoedema or will be diagnosed with lymphoedema in the future. The idea was a single website featuring salient information and introducing you to the medical experts, the product providers, the professional organisations, the charities, the support groups and other people living with lymphoedema, all in one place. I wanted this website to be free of charge for people to join as a member and then receive exclusive membership benefits. I also wanted to donate 25% of pre-tax profits to lymphoedema charities.

I had the concept, now I needed a suitable brand name. Lymphoedema United captured everything I wanted my website and company to be. My aim is to unite people suffering from the disease, with all the key contacts from the lymphoedema community. I decided to write this book to share my experiences and helpful tips to mark my 10-year lymphaversary on 19th June 2021. The website will keep you up to date with current news and future developments. I am thrilled that most of the wonderful people who have written in this book are also featuring on my website *www.lymphoedemaunited.com*, in particular on the Meet the Experts panel.

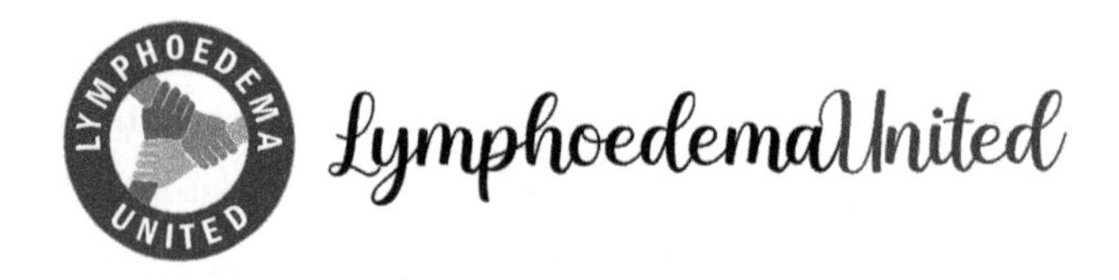

Alongside the website will be a presence on various social media platforms like Facebook, Twitter, LinkedIn, Instagram and YouTube. This will be under the abbreviated and more international-friendly brand name of LymphUnited. This allows me to instantly communicate breaking news and important messages to the lymphoedema community following me.

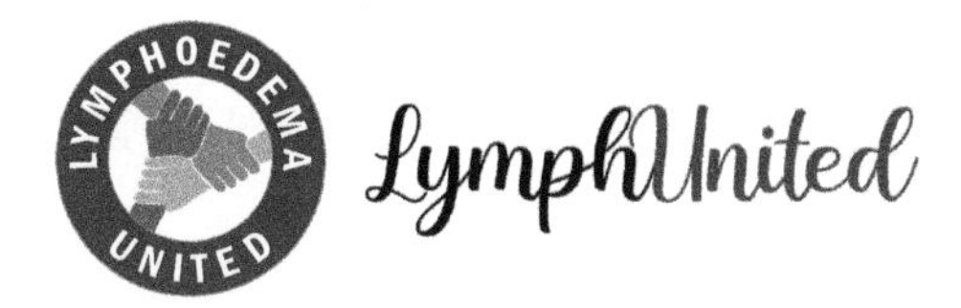

LymphUnited will also be the name of the quarterly eNewsletter, exclusive to those who have signed up as a free member of LymphoedemaUnited.com.

The final part of this project will be to launch LymphUnited as a Lymphoedema Support Group on Facebook, to help people with the condition to find others who will understand, encouraging us to talk more, listen to others who need reassurance and share tips on how we can live better with lymphoedema.

Top Tip #40: Sign up now as a Free Member of *www.lymphoedemaunited.com* and follow us on social media using @LymphUnited.

27

CONCLUSION

Lymphoedema is a chronic life-changing disease that can have an enormous detrimental effect on your physical and mental health. It can create despair and loneliness, pain and embarrassment, and a feeling of being isolated and lost, not knowing where or who to turn to for help. Whilst writing this book I have been told that in some cases, it can be life-threatening.

Lymphoedema is a disease that continually struggles to be heard above the justifiably powerful noise of more familiar life-threatening diseases, that may well have taken the life of someone we know.

Encouragingly, with the continued efforts of the lymphoedema community, awareness of this chronic lifelong disease is increasing. Comprehensive information is now easily accessible, training modules have improved knowledge, especially in the General Practitioner sector, resulting in more people being correctly diagnosed with lymphoedema. Of course, once we know what the problem is, then we can aim to solve it, or in the case of lymphoedema, manage it, until such time as a cure is found.

Once diagnosed, the next crucial step is to find a local, qualified and experienced lymphoedema therapist, trained to perform Decongestive Lymphatic Therapy including Manual Lymphatic Drainage. If you are lucky enough to find such a therapist on the NHS, they will provide physical and mental support for many years to come. Not only will they understand the many challenges you will face by having lymphoedema; they will also recommend solutions to improve your quality of life. For example, by measuring and arranging the supply of properly fitted compression garments and products, with the aim of reducing and maintaining the swelling. In addition, your lymphoedema therapist should also inform you and teach you self-management techniques, helping you to control the swelling whilst away from the clinic. Put simply, they will be your trusted co-pilot and knowledgeable navigator during your journey with lymphoedema. Tell them absolutely everything.

Once informed or taught about the four cornerstones of good self-management (Skin Care, Compression, Healthy Lifestyle & Movement and Lymphatic Drainage), it is up to us to look after ourselves physically and apply these disciplines on a daily, if not regular, basis.

Of course, the other battle with lymphoedema is to look after your mental wellbeing and find someone to talk with, who understands your circumstances. Social media allows you to be vocal and visible, or informed and invisible, or a combination of them all. With several online support groups operating on Facebook, you can join a lymphoedema community of like-minded people who are seeking help and guidance and who can also share their personal experiences with others. Remember, you are not alone and it's good to talk. There is also the telephone helpline at the Lymphoedema Support Network, if you would prefer a one-on-one conversation.

Knowledge is power and there is a wealth of information accessible both online on websites, blogs and newsletters, plus paper leaflets from some organisations if preferred, and some excellent books. If we can educate ourselves about lymphoedema using the material available to us, then we can better understand the condition and how we can manage it more effectively.

One of the positives about lymphoedema is that it's a niche sector. If, and when, you are in a better place, you may choose to make a worthy contribution to the lymphoedema community. No matter how large or small, *you really can make a difference.* Whether that's fundraising or volunteering for one of the lymphoedema charities, raising awareness of lymphoedema with your local GPs by taking in leaflets or posters, or joining a support group and sharing your tips and experiences, it all helps. Positive Mental Attitude is there in all of us, but sometimes it takes a while to believe in yourself, increase confidence and self-esteem. For me, finding clothes that made me look 'normal' again, provided the confidence boost I needed to come out of my shell and walk tall again.

As Professor Mortimer so passionately explained, money will attract medical scientists to conduct research, with the aim of finding a cure for lymphoedema. If 25% of the 450,000 people with lymphoedema in the UK raised £25, that would provide over £2.8m to help fund medical research. That's an extraordinary example of what we could do if we all pulled together.

Until a cure is found, if the usual treatments and therapies are not effective in reducing and maintaining your swelling, then perhaps discuss the various surgeries that are available with your therapist or GP. Investigations that may well include a lymphoscintigraphy, could ascertain whether lymph node transfer, lymphovenous anastomosis and/or liposuction are suitable options for you.

Thank you for purchasing and taking the time to read my book. I sincerely hope that you are doing OK and that this book has given you a handful of tips to help you to live better with lymphoedema. Please get in touch and unite with the lymphoedema community as a free member of *www.lymphoedemaunited.com* and opt in to receive the quarterly newsletter and bulletins.

AFTERWORD

So, how am I doing now? I have had all the surgery that is suitable for my condition and the liposuction was very successful, reducing my leg volume considerably. However, I cannot be complacent, as I still have a fear of rebound. Due to taking up cycling to help with my fitness, my calf has increased in size and my thigh has reduced, albeit with a bit more muscle than before. Therefore, my lower leg is almost the same circumference now as my upper leg, which I try not to be too disheartened about. The easiest thing I do to snap myself out of any hint of negativity, is to look at the photo of my leg in 2011 and compare it to my leg now. It is much improved, as is my confidence and self-esteem. I recognise that I am one of the lucky ones, for which I am immensely grateful.

Is it incredibly good planning, or just coincidence, that I write this penultimate paragraph of my book on 19th June 2021, exactly 10 years to the day when I fell poorly with cellulitis that led to my lymphoedema? I cannot imagine that the next 10 years will be as much of a rollercoaster as the previous decade turned out to be. Having now exhausted all avenues available, I believe it's now up to me to try and maintain the current size and prevent further rebound.

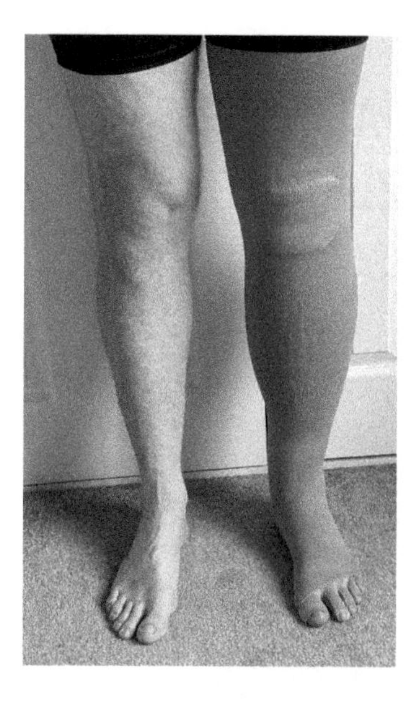

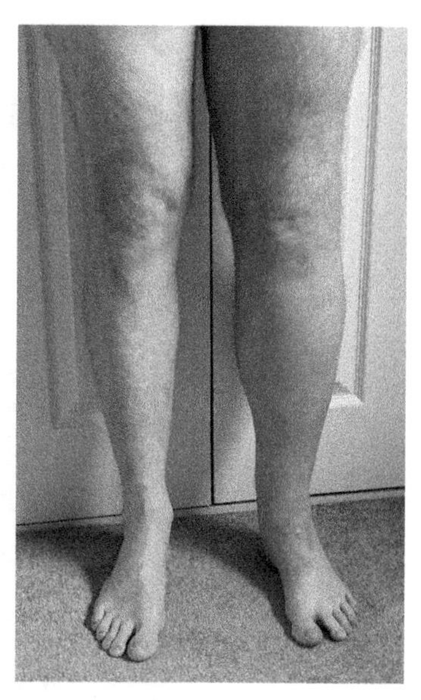

Matt's legs on 19th June 2021, exactly 10 years with lymphoedema

If I am still around when a cure is found, then great, put my name down for it. In the meantime, my objective is to control the swelling, ideally reducing the volume through better lifestyle choices and exercise whilst maintaining a Positive Mental Attitude. 20th June 2021, my Father's Day gift from my wife and daughter, a Fitbit. Now there is no excuse for me not to keep moving!

I hope that my book does, in some small way, help others to *live better with lymphoedema*.

Please remember:
You are not alone.
Control your lymphoedema, don't let your lymphoedema control you.
Stay Positive, Keep Talking, Make a Difference

MEET THE AUTHOR
MATT HAZLEDINE

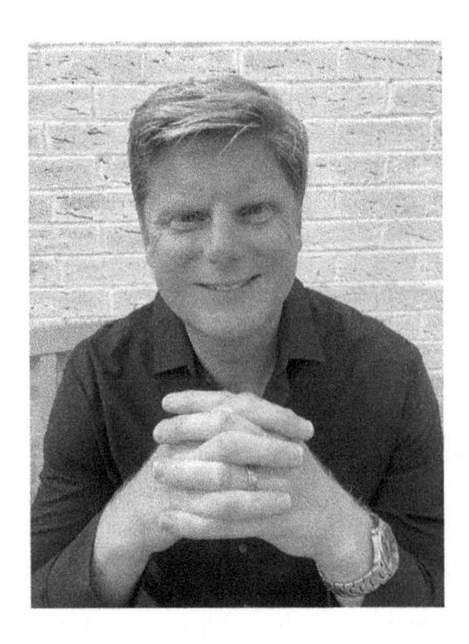

In 2011, at the age of 40, Matt experienced a severe episode of cellulitis in his left leg, which hospitalised him for 13 nights. This subsequently caused a significant swelling called lymphoedema, a chronic lifelong disease with no cure.

In 2021, to commemorate 10 years of living with this life-changing condition, he wrote this book to share his extensive experiences and useful tips to help other people to live better with lymphoedema.

Matt invited a couple of medical professionals, whom he has been a patient of since 2012, to contribute some invaluable information and trusted guidance about lymphoedema. Both Professor Mortimer and Dr Gordon instantly agreed and so he continued to ask all the other wonderful people who have been involved in his journey to feature in his book. Nobody said no.

Whether you are newly diagnosed with lymphoedema or have had the condition for some time, this book will provide beneficial suggestions on the most salient subjects. In the first couple of years with lymphoedema, Matt really struggled to come to terms with adjusting his life to accommodate his very swollen leg. Through trial and error, he has worn every appropriate compression garment, tested almost every product, had all therapies known to him and two different types of surgery. He now knows what works for him and what doesn't. He shares these trials and tribulations to inform you of what products and services out there to assist you and who to go to for help.

Over the past few years, he has been in a much happier and positive place and has continued his mission to help others living with the condition, whilst raising money for lymphoedema charities. Matt has been a Trustee of the Lymphoedema Support Network, featured in the Health Section of the Daily Mail, written for newsletters, blogs and books, been interviewed on local hospital radio and so far, raised nearly £20,000 for various charities.

He is a family man, who enjoys reading, playing golf, supporting Southend United and socialising with close friends. Matt is motivated to make a positive difference and help others to live better with lymphoedema.

If you would like to get in touch with Matt, please send him a message via his website *www.lymphoedemaunited.com* and follow him on Facebook and Twitter using @LymphUnited.

ACKNOWLEDGEMENTS

I would like to take this opportunity to thank the following incredible and selfless people in the lymphoedema sector, for the positive impact that they have had on my life and for sharing some of their extensive knowledge of lymphoedema in my book:

Professor Peter Mortimer
Professor Dominic Furniss
Professor Christine Moffatt
Professor Vaughan Keeley
Dr Kristiana Gordon
Patryk Gawrysiak
Mark Pearson
Kelly Nickson
Rebecca Elwell
Jane Wigg
Anita Wallace
Margaret Sneddon
Carol Ellis
William Repicci
Gaynor Leech
Tom Wright
Naomi Northen-Ellis
Julian Pearce
Elizabeth Radcliffe
Clare Anvar
Sally Kay
Gemma Levine
Amerjit Chohan

I would like to say a special, heartfelt thank you to Professor Peter Mortimer for his care and for writing the Foreword for my book. He has willingly given his support and encouragement to my projects.

May I also thank my wife, Vicki and dear friends Vikki Vellacott and Jo Copper, plus my new friend Mel, for reading my draft copy and providing their honest and constructive opinions.

With thanks to my publisher, Wordzworth. In particular, Doug Morris, Kelly Roche and the design team for their professional and helpful advice and for bringing my book to the lymphoedema community in the UK, USA, Australia and Europe. Thank you.

DONATIONS

I always planned to self-fund the publication of my book. However, I would like to thank Tom Wright from Haddenham Healthcare Ltd and Naomi Northen-Ellis from Compression Therapy UK Ltd for their generous donations, which have helped towards the publishing costs.

APPENDIX I
SUMMARY OF THE 'TOP TIPS' FOR YOUR WALL

I hope that you have found my Top Tips helpful. I thought it might be useful to put them all in one area, so if you choose to, you can cut these pages out and put them somewhere visible as a constant reminder to help you to live better with lymphoedema.

Finding the right therapist

Top Tip #1: If diagnosed with lymphoedema, get a referral from your GP to a qualified therapist as soon as possible.

Top Tip #2: To find your nearest qualified lymphoedema therapist, visit *www.thebls.com/directory*

Mental Wellbeing and Support Groups

Top Tip #3: Write a Gratitude List of 3 things that you are grateful for every day. Say them to yourself in the mirror every morning. Go on, give it a try, nothing to lose, right?

Top Tip #4: Get some fresh air, go for a walk and appreciate your natural surroundings. Nature is calming and therapeutic.

Top Tip #5: Connect with other people with lymphoedema by joining online support groups. Also, try to meet others in person at local support group meetings. Ask your therapist for information.

Top Tip #6: Visit patient-based websites and sign up for newsletters and/or join as a free member: LymphoedemaUnited.com, Legs Matter.org, Lymph-what-oedema.com and legclub.org

Top Tip #7: Become a member of the LSN. It's a must for anyone with lymphoedema. Website: *lymphoedema.org* Email: *admin@lsn.org.uk* Telephone: *020 7351 4480* or *020 7351 0990*

Compression Garments, Products & Aids

Top Tip #8: Shop around for durable rubber gloves to assist donning. There is no need to pay over £2 per pair.

Top Tip #9: Research products available from specialist lymphoedema suppliers' websites and discuss them with your therapist or GP to find out whether they are suitable for you.

Top Tip #10: If your compression garment is causing pain or numbness, or discomfort, is too tight, too loose, not fitting correctly in any way, speak to your therapist as a priority.

Top Tip #11: Take your old compression garments on holiday and wear them when you are swimming or sunbathing.

Top Tip #12: Only get your compression garments measured by a qualified and experienced lymphoedema therapist.

Cellulitis

Top Tip #13: Photocopy the *Management of Cellulitis Guidance* section and ask your GP to add it to your file. Also put a copy in your Medical Emergency Pack just in case you experience symptoms of cellulitis in future.

Top Tip #14: Produce a Medical Emergency Pack, just in case you get cellulitis symptoms in future.

Skin Care

Top Tip #15: Evaluate any sports or hobbies you enjoy, that could put you at risk of damaging or breaking your skin.

Top Tip #16: Perform a risk assessment at your workplace and put steps in place to reduce the risk of damaging or breaking your skin, getting an infection.

Top Tip #17: Sign up for an annual NHS Prescription Prepayment Certificate and save money (if usual prescription costs apply to you, of course). *https://www.nhsbsa.nhs.uk/help-nhs-prescription-costs/prescription-prepayment-certificates-ppcs*

Top Tip #18: Don't ever run out of skin care products! When down to the last three shower emollients, tear off the lid of the box as a reminder to order a repeat prescription.

Top Tip #19: Put a sticky note on the skin care guidance page, for ease of reference.

Healthy Lifestyle

Top Tip #20: Calculate and monitor your own Body Mass Index (BMI) using the calculator on the NHS Live Well website. The considered healthy BMI is between 18.5 and 24.9. *https://www.nhs.uk/live-well/healthy-weight/bmi-calculator/*

Top Tip #21: Set an alarm on your phone for every 30 minutes throughout the day as a reminder to get up and move about. Alternatively, invest in a Fitbit which monitors your movement automatically.

Top Tip #22: Ask your lymphoedema therapist for information on the types of movement or light exercise that are particularly suitable for your personal circumstances.

Top Tip #23: If you do fancy an unhealthy treat, limit the portion size or quantity to help you to maintain a healthy weight.

Top Tip #24: Produce a line graph in Excel and record your weight every month. It's an instant visual guide on weight loss and gain.

Top Tip #25: Identify your weak spots, eg: certain times of day or triggers when you are more likely to eat unhealthy snacks or foods and change the routine. Fill that time with another distraction or swap the snack for something that is less bad for you.

Top Tip #26: When watching TV, stand up and do some stretches every time the adverts come on, or if you find it difficult to stand, stretch out your legs and rotate your ankles in both directions.

Top Tip #27: Purchase a water beaker with time markers on to motivate you to drink the right amount of water or fluid per day.

Top Tip #28: Assign 3 days of the week when you do not drink alcohol, preferably together, eg: Monday to Wednesday.

Top Tip #29: Limit alcohol consumption on Thursday and Sunday as, typically, weekend consumption is higher.

Top Tip #39: Purchase a Thera Band and use it as part of your daily movement and exercise, in the comfort of your own home. Check out YouTube for instructional videos.

Decongestive Lymphatic Therapy

Top Tip #30: Talk to your Lymphoedema Therapist or GP about arranging Decongestive Lymphatic Therapy (DLT), if you haven't already.

Top Tip #31: Try to avoid having Multi-Layer Lymphoedema Bandaging (MLLB) during hot weather to try and prevent folliculitis. Check the long-range weather forecast for your area on the Met Office website *www.metoffice,gov.uk*.

Top Tip #32: Measure your limb monthly and record on an Excel line graph. If you see any increase in size, use a compression wrap system to try and reduce the volume. However, if you experience a constant increase in size, please contact your lymphoedema therapist for advice.

Top Tip #33: If you work at a desk for long periods, invest in a comfortable foot stool on wheels, that is the right height to elevate your leg, comfortably, under your desk.

Top Tip #34: Ask your therapist or GP to prescribe appropriately sized Compression Wrap System to use when you experience increased swelling.

Top Tip #38: Investigate whether a Compression Pump works for you, by arranging a two-week trial free of charge.

Clothes and Shoes:

Top Tip #35: Put yourself first. Remember *"in the event of an emergency, pull down and apply your own oxygen mask first before helping others."*

Top Tip #36: To justify the cost of buying bespoke clothes or shoes, calculate the cost divided by the number of times you will wear it = 'cost per wear.' Then apply increased self-esteem, greater confidence, feeling great, looking good.....shall I go on?

Top Tip #37: Invest in yourself and improve your mental wellbeing by purchasing perfectly fitting made-to-measure clothes and shoes.

Free Membership Website - Many Members' Benefits available

Top Tip #40: Sign up now as a Free Member of *www.lymphoedemaunited.com* and follow us on social media using @LymphUnited.

APPENDIX II
CHARITY FUNDRAISING & DONATIONS

You can support lymphoedema charities and organisations in raising money by arranging a fundraising event or simply by making a donation. Any amount of money that you donate will make a positive difference to the lymphoedema community and assist these charities and organisations to continue their excellent work in helping people living with lymphoedema.

Lymphoedema Research Fund

https://www.stgeorgeshospitalcharity.org.uk/donate/intro

The British Lymphology Society (BLS)

https://www.thebls.com/pages/support-us

The Lymphoedema Support Network (LSN)

https://www.lymphoedema.org/get-involved/make-a-donation
https://www.lymphoedema.org/get-involved/fundraising

MLD UK

http://www.mlduk.org.uk/lymfund/

Lymphatic Education & Research Network (LE&RN)

https://lymphaticnetwork.org/get-involved/donate
https://lymphaticnetwork.org/supporting-member

International Lymphoedema Framework (ILF)

https://www.lympho.org/please-donate

APPENDIX III
RESOURCES: USEFUL LINKS, BOOKS & WEBSITES

Patient Based Websites

www.lymphoedemaunited.com
www.lymphodema.org.
www.legsmatter.com
www.legclub.org
www.lymph-what-oedema.com
www.lwocommunity4families.com

Lymphoedema Support Groups

LymphUnited
HealthUnlocked
www.facebook.com/groups/LWOSupportGroup
www.facebook.com/groups/lwocommunity4families

Lymphoedema Organisations and Charities

www.thebls.com The British Lymphology Society (BLS)
www.lymphoedema.org The Lymphoedema Support Network (LSN)
www.mlduk.org.uk MLD UK
www.lymphaticnetwork.org Lymphatic Education & Research Network (LE&RN)
www.lympho.org International Lymphoedema Framework (ILF)
www.stgeorgeshospitalcharity.org.uk Lymphoedema Research Fund

Lymphoedema Directories for Therapists & Specialists

Directories

www.thebls.com/directory
www.mlduk.org.uk/therapists
www.lymphaticnetwork.org/centers-of-excellence

Specialists

www.reflexologylymphdrainage.co.uk
www.lymphvision.com
www.olp.surgery

NHS - Useful Links

www.nhs.uk/conditions/cellulitis/
www.nhs.uk/mental-health/self-help
www.nhs.uk/live-well
www.nhs.uk/live-well/eat-well
https://www.nhs.uk/better-health/quit-smoking/
www.nhs.uk/live-well/healthy-weight/bmi-calculator/
www.nhsbsa.nhs.uk/help-nhs-prescription-costs/prescription-prepayment-certificates-ppcs

Specialist Companies, Useful Products and Online Shops

www.compressiontherapyuk.com
www.lymphshop.com by Haddenham Healthcare Ltd
www.sieden.co.uk
www.mediuk.co.uk/shop by Medi UK Ltd
www.sigvaris.com/en-gb Sigvaris UK
www.shop.lrselfcare.co.uk by L&R Medical UK Ltd
www.healthandcare.co.uk (type 'lymphoedema' into their search tool)

www.daylong.co.uk by Credenhill Ltd
www.charlies.co.uk Gloves

Clothes and Shoes

www.levi.com
www.dress2kill.com
www.itailor.com
www.itailor.com/collection/women/
www.itailorshoes.com
www.hotter.com
www.widefitshoes.co.uk
www.cosyfeet.com
www.skechers.com
www.clarks.co.uk.
www.softtopsocks.co.uk
www.hj.co.uk/softtop
www.sockshop.co.uk/
www.socksnob.co.uk/
www.bambooclothing.co.uk.

Other Useful Contacts

www.samaritans.org
www.macmillan.org.uk
www.lipoedema.co.uk

Reports and Documents by Medical Professionals

"Cellulitis in chronic oedema of the lower leg: an international cross-sectional study." available on *www.onlinelibrary.wiley.com.*

Cellulitis guidance

www.lymphoedema.org/wp-content/uploads/2020/01/cellulitis_consensus.pdf

COVID vaccination guidance

www.lymphoedema.org/wp-content/uploads/2021/02/Consensus_Document_on_COVID_Vaccination_12feb2021.pdf

Books

Let's Talk Lymphoedema by Professor Peter Mortimer and Gemma Levine
Lymphedema and Lipedema Nutrition Guide by Ehrlich, Iker, Herbst, Kahn, Sears, Kenyon, McMahon
The Complete Lymphedema Management and Nutrition Guide by Jean Lamantia and Ann Dimenna
Covid Thoughts by Gemma Levine
Aqua by Gemma Levine

APPENDIX IV
REFERENCES

Chapter 3 What is Primary Lymphoedema?

References

A new classification system for primary lymphatic dysplasias based on phenotype.
Connell F, Brice G, Jeffery S, Keeley V, Mortimer P, Mansour S.
Clinical Genetics 2010; 77(5):438-52.

Lymphoedema: an underestimated health problem.
Moffatt CJ, Franks PJ, Doherty DC, et al.
Q J Med 2003; 96: 731–8.

Update and audit of the St George's classification algorithm of primary lymphatic anomalies: a clinical and molecular approach to diagnosis.
Gordon K, Varney R, Keeley V, Riches K, Jeffery S, Van Zanten M, Mortimer P, Ostergaard P, Mansour S.
Journal of Medical Genetics 2020; 57(10):653-659.

Chapter 4 How common is Chronic Oedema?

References

Moffatt C.J., Keeley V, Quéré I. (2019). 'The Concept of Chronic Edema-A Neglected Public Health Issue and an International Response: The LIMPRINT Study' *Lymphat Res Biol*; 17(2): 121-126. doi: 10.1089/lrb.2018.0085.

Schulze H., Nacke M., Gutenbrunner C. and Hadamitzky C. (2018). 'Worldwide assessment of healthcare personnel dealing with lymphoedema' *Health economics review*; 8(1): 10. *https://doi.org/10.1186/s13561-018-0194-6*

WHO (2021). *Lymphatic filariasis*. Available at: *https://www.who.int/lymphatic_filariasis/epidemiology/en/#:~:text=An%20estimated%20120%20million%20people,or%20elephantiasis%20of%20the%20leg*. [Accessed on 20th April 2021]

Moffatt C.J., Franks P.J., Doherty D.C., Williams A.F., Badger C., Jeffs E., Bosanquet N. and Mortimer P.S. (2003). 'Lymphoedema: an underestimated health problem' *Q J Med*; 96: 731-438.

Moffatt C.J., Keeley V., Franks P.J., Rich A. and Pinnington L.L. (2016). 'Chronic oedema: a prevalent health care problem for UK health services' *International Wound Journal*; 14(5): 772-781.

Parliament UK (2014). *Health Committee: Written evidence from the Lymphoedema Support Network (LTC 10)*. Available at: *https://publications.parliament.uk/pa/cm201415/cmselect/cmhealth/401/401vw09.htm* [Accessed on 20th April 2021]

The Scottish Government & Macmillan Cancer Support (2013). *Lymphoedema Care in Scotland: Achieving Equity and Quality*. Edinburgh: The Scottish Government. Available at:

https://www.gov.scot/binaries/content/documents/govscot/publications/independent-report/2013/11/smasac-short-life-working-group-lymphoedema-lymphoedema-care-scotland-achieving-equity-quality/documents/lymphoedema-care-scotland-achieving-equity-quality/lymphoedema-care-scotland-achieving-equity-quality/govscot%3Adocument/00438797.pdf [Accessed on 18th April 2021]

CREST (2008). *Guidelines for The Diagnosis, Assessment and Management of Lymphoedema*. Belfast: CREST Secretariat. Available at: *Https://Www.Lymphoedemasupportni.Org/Sites/Default/Files/Crest_Guidelines_On_The_Diagnosis__Assessment_And_Management_Of_Lymphoedema.Pdf* [Accessed on 18th April 2021]

Lymphoedema Network Wales (2021). *Lymphoedema Network Wales Annual Report 2020-2021*. Unpublished.

ONS (2020). *Population estimates for the UK, England and Wales, Scotland and Northern Ireland: mid-2019*. Available at: *https://www.ons.gov.uk/peoplepopulationandcommunity/populationandmigration/populationestimates/bulletins/annualmidyearpopulationestimates/mid2019estimates* [Accessed on 11th May 2021]

[11]Moffatt C.J., Gaskin R., Sykorova M., Dring E., Aubeeluck A., Franks P.J., Windrum P., Mercier G., Pinnington L and Quéré, I (2019). 'Prevalence and Risk Factors for Chronic Edema in U.K. Community Nursing Services' *Lymphatic Research and Biology. 17*(2): 147-154. *https://doi.org/10.1089/lrb.2018.0086*

Quéré I., Palmier S., Noerregaard S., Pastor J., Sykorova M., Dring E., Franks P. J., Murray S., Keeley V., Bermark S., Karlsmark T., Kyne N., Colgan M. P., Coulombe M. M., Mestre S., Mercier G., & Moffatt C. J. (2019). 'LIMPRINT: Estimation of the Prevalence of Lymphoedema/Chronic Oedema in Acute Hospital in In-Patients' *Lymphatic research and biology, 17*(2): 135–140. *https://doi.org/10.1089/lrb.2019.0024*

Moffatt C.J., Sykorova M., Aubeeluck A., Franks P.J., Pankhurst S., Bussey R., Whiston S., Murray S., Mercier G., Quere I. and Gordon S. (2019). 'Clinical and Ethical Challenges in Undertaking LIMPRINT in Vulnerable Populations' *Lymphatic Research and Biology*. 17(2): 155-162.

[4] Moffatt C.J. and Pinnington L. (2012). 'Facilitating Development of Community Based Lymphoedema Services Through Clinical Education' *Project Evaluation Report*. University of Nottingham and Derby Hospitals NHS Trust, Nottingham.

[5] Moffatt C.J., Keeley V., Franks P.J., Rich A. and Pinnington L.L. (2016). 'Chronic oedema: a prevalent health care problem for UK health services' *International Wound Journal*; 14(5): 772-781.

[6] Cooper G. and Bagnall A. (2016). 'Prevalence of lymphoedema in the UK: focus on the Southwest and West Midlands' *British Journal of Community Nursing*; Chronic Oedema Suppl:S6-14.

[17]Moffatt C.J., Keeley V., Franks P.J., Rich A. and Pinnington L.L. (2016). 'Chronic oedema: a prevalent health care problem for UK health services' *International Wound Journal*; 14(5): 772-781.

[8] Moffatt C.J., Keeley V., Franks P.J., Rich A. and Pinnington L.L. (2016). 'Chronic oedema: a prevalent health care problem for UK health services' *International Wound Journal*; 14(5): 772-781.

[19] Burian E.A., *Karlsmark* T., Franks P.J., Keeley V., *Quéré* I. and Moffatt C.J. (2021). 'Cellulitis in chronic oedema of the lower leg: an international cross-sectional study' *British Journal of Dermatology*. Online ahead of print. *https://doi.org/10.1111/bjd.19803*

[20] Greene A.K., *Zurakowski* D. and *Goss* J.A. (2020). 'Body Mass Index and Lymphedema Morbidity: Comparison of Obese versus Normal-Weight Patients' *Plast Reconstr Surg*;146(2): 402-407.

[21] Cooper G. (2013). 'Lymphoedema prevalence in the West Midlands region' *Journal of Lymphoedema*; 8(1): 17-20.

[22] Keast D., Moffatt C. and *Janmohammad* A. (2019). 'Lymphedema Impact and Prevalence International Study: The Canadian Data' *Lymphatic Research and Biology*; *17(2)*: 178-186. *https://doi.org/10.1089/lrb.2019.0014*

[23] Parliament UK (2014). *Health Committee: Written evidence from the Lymphoedema Support Network (LTC 10)*. Available at: *https://publications.parliament.uk/pa/cm201415/cmselect/cmhealth/401/401vw09.htm* [Accessed on 20th April 2021]

[24] NHS (2019). *Overview: Lymphoedema*. Available at: *https://www.nhs.uk/conditions/lymphoedema/#:~:text=Lymphoedema%20is%20thought%20to%20affect,lymphoedema%20is%20much%20more%20common* [Accessed on 25th April 2021]

[25] Cooper G. and Bagnall A. (2016). 'Prevalence of lymphoedema in the UK: focus on the Southwest and West Midlands' *British Journal of Community Nursing*; Chronic Oedema Suppl:S6-14.

[26] Moffatt C.J., Keeley V, Quéré I. (2019). 'The Concept of Chronic Edema-A Neglected Public Health Issue and an International Response: The LIMPRINT Study' *Lymphat Res Biol*; 17(2): 121-126. doi: 10.1089/lrb.2018.0085.

[27] Cancer Research UK (2020). *Lymphoedema after breast cancer treatment.* Available at: *https://www.cancerresearchuk.org/about-cancer/breast-cancer/living-with/lymphoedema-after-treatment* [Accessed on 25th April 2021]

[28] NHS (2019). *Overview: Lymphoedema.* Available at: *https://www.nhs.uk/conditions/lymphoedema/#:~:text=Lymphoedema%20is%20thought%20to%20affect,lymphoedema%20is%20much%20more%20common* [Accessed on 25th April 2021]

[29] Whayman N. (2015). 'The causes and treatment of wet weeping legs' *Wound Essentials*; 10(1): 30-34.

[30] Dowsett C., Bielby A. and Searle R. (2014). 'Reconciling increasing wound care demands with available resources' *J Wound Care*; 23(11): 552, 554, 556-8 passim. doi: 10.12968/jowc.2014.23.11.552.

Chapter 14 Lymphatic Drainage Techniques & Kinesiology Tape

References

Foldi, M., Foldi, E., 2012. Földi's Textbook of Lymphology for Physicians and Lymphedema Therapists. 3rd Ed. New York, Elsevier.

Zuther, J., and Norton, S., 2018. Lymphedem Management, The Comprehensive Guide for Practitioners. Fourth Ed. New York, Thieme Medical Publishers

Lightning Source UK Ltd.
Milton Keynes UK
UKHW021833081021
391866UK00007B/326

9 781783 24220